GET YOUR MOJO BACK

Sex, Pleasure and Intimacy
After Birth

CLIO WOOD

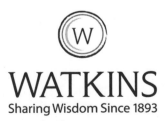

WATKINS
Sharing Wisdom Since 1893

Get Your Mojo Back
Clio Wood

First published in the UK and USA in 2023 by
Watkins, an imprint of Watkins Media Limited
Unit 11, Shepperton House, 83–93 Shepperton Road
London N1 3DF

enquiries@watkinspublishing.com

Commissioning Editor: Anya Hayes
Senior Editor: Lucy Carroll
Assistant Editor: Brittany Willis
Head of Design: Karen Smith
Illustrator: Sneha Alexander
Illustration concept on page 6: Clio Wood
Production: Uzma Taj

A CIP record for this book is available from the British Library

ISBN: 978-1-78678-695-1 (Paperback)
ISBN: 978-1-78678-695-5 (eBook)

10 9 8 7 6 5 4 3 2 1

Printed in United Kingdom by TJ Books Limited

www.watkinspublishing.com

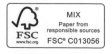

For my past, present and future selves and
the journey we're on; and for my beautiful family,
B, D & E, without whom I wouldn't be where I am

CONTENTS

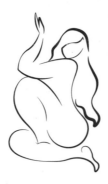

ABOUT THE AUTHOR

I am Clio Wood, women's health & sex positivity advocate and Founder of &breathe, an award-winning family wellbeing company supporting pre- and post-natal women, families and women in the perimenopause period. I created &Breathe in 2015, following the traumatic birth of my daughter in 2014. I suffered postnatal depression as well as mild post-traumatic stress disorder (PTSD), a too-tight pelvic floor and painful sex. This all contributed to marriage problems which nearly ended in divorce. I struggled to find the support I needed as a new parent, and wanted to help other women be their best selves through fitness, food and feeling good, so I started &Breathe.

My work as an advocate, writer and speaker has grown naturally from my own experience of mental health and physical (pelvic floor) issues postnatally, as well as my work with retreat and event guests and by creating our expert &Breathe team. It has underlined what I've always known: that sex, intimacy and relationships (particularly postnatally, but beyond this and into parenthood too) are a key part of our life experience. They make up a good deal of our fears and worries, but we're not just talking about them.

I have written for the *Telegraph*, *I. Paper*, *HuffPost*, *Mother & Baby* and *Motherdom Magazine* and spoken on numerous podcasts such as *The Parent Hood* with Marina Fogle, *Breaking Mum & Dad* with Anna Williamson and *Motherkind* with Zoe Blaskey.

I live in East London with my husband, Bryn, and our two daughters, Delphi and Echo. I love unusual names, ice cream, keeping strong, reading and finding new places.

Find out more: www.andbreathewellbeing.com | on Instagram @andbreathewellbeing and @itscliowood

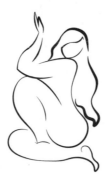

INTRODUCTION

What do 83 per cent of new mothers have in common, apart from wanting to sell their own offspring for an hour's sleep?[1] Bingo. It's that they're all going through some form of sexual dysfunction and pain. I made up the bit about sleep (though I'm betting I'm pretty close), but the sexual dysfunction study is for real.

I'm Clio, and I'm one of that 83 per cent. It's hard not to be. You might be too. And if not, you certainly know someone who is, whether or not they've told you about it. I had a traumatic birth experience which, when layered onto my existing depression and insecurity (hello, inner critic!), meant that my postnatal experience was more than a small shock to the system. I suffered postnatal depression and spent my days crying, raging and more. I struggled with painful breastfeeding, and I had a total loss of identity and felt completely at odds with my husband.

I thought at least that my postnatal fitness journey wouldn't be a problem. I was always sporty through school and university, and keeping fit and active is an important part of my life and mental health. I was so keen to keep my pelvic floor toned and tight that I went into Kegel overdrive, doing pelvic floor exercises whenever I could during pregnancy. That wasn't the right approach, as it turns out, because I hadn't been taught properly how to do a pelvic floor lift (also called a Kegel, after Arnold Kegel, an American gynaecologist), and this led to a pelvic floor that was *too* tight. The combination of my depression and uncertainty, which made my entire body tense, from my shoulders to my toes, and vaginal scarring meant sex became practically impossible.

Sadly, all of this is far too common. But the thing is: Common. Does. Not. Mean. Normal. Just because lots of people experience something doesn't mean that's how it should be. So my question is, if so many of us are suffering, why aren't we talking about it more? Why do we feel weird about bringing it up with our friends, let alone our doctors? The 83 per cent statistic is such a high figure: if this huge percentage of us at three months postnatal are cringing at the thought of intimacy with their other half, shouldn't more of us be looking for answers? If enough of us are asking . . . well, *are* enough of us asking?

Okay, so three months postnatal is pretty soon for most of us to be jumping back in the sack, and perhaps too soon to be expecting a flourishing sex life again. You have, after all, pushed an actual human being out of your vagina, or undergone major abdominal surgery. But what would you say if, crawling forward to six months postpartum, the figure experiencing painful sex and sexual dysfunction reduces only slightly, to 64 per cent?[2]

You're probably still sleep deprived, though getting into the swing of parenthood; you might develop, or still have, postnatal depression or other mood disorder; you're probably nervous about your core and pelvic floor, even if your rehabilitation has gone smoothly; you'll soon be on to weaning and thinking ahead to childcare if you plan to return to work outside the home. At least your baby might be moving out of your bedroom, but it's not all smooth sailing from here! Family life is full on. Where do you find the time to even *think about*, let alone *improve* your sex life?

The first year of parenthood is the time when marriage satisfaction rates are the lowest,[3] but what about later in parenthood, when lack of sleep is no longer the main issue, and you don't hate your partner quite so much? Added to that, what happens when your sex drive dries up and intimacy doesn't bring you pleasure any more? Maybe you think that's something you just have to live with, but what if you don't?

Having a baby, however it comes out, is a big experience. It might have been wonderful, soulful and healing. It might have been exactly the opposite, as mine was. But whatever your experience, it becomes part of your identity. And it *changes* your identity as a woman, including your sexual identity. This book is not just about the postnatal period, though the way that you are empowered, or not, to deal with intimacy in that time is key, but about sex after birth as the gateway to intimacy for the rest of your life. Once postnatal, always postnatal. Let's make sure that pleasure is part of the equation too.

It might not be easy, but I want to help. Because although you're not talking about it, I know you want to hear that others are going through the same thing. Whenever the subject of sex comes up, in whispered conversations, at events, on our retreats, with my friends, I see the relief on your faces when you realise you're not alone. I know from the messages I receive that you want to talk, to ask questions and to feel supported.

My own experience of postnatal sex first time round was painful and emotional, but ultimately the long journey I've been on has had a positive and happy outcome. I felt alone, and was made to feel ignorant at many points along the way. I had to fight to receive the care I needed, digging deep to find the answers that should have been clearly signposted from the beginning, and I want others to find their solution more quickly. I don't want others to suffer (for themselves or in their relationship) as I did. I want *you* to learn from the mistakes that *I* experienced.

My experience is a conventional, heterosexual, cis-gendered one, and I write with that in mind. There are, of course, many different types of families out there – from single mothers, to adoptive couples, to same-sex partnerships. I hope that my book, as well as its information and the cause that it champions, extends to these other set-ups despite being centred on my own journey.

So welcome to *Get Your Mojo Back*. Because a) it's totally possible, even if it doesn't feel like it now, and b) no-one else is giving it to you straight. Read this book. Check out the further reading at the end of each chapter, and the resources listed at the end of the book and on www.andbreathewellbeing.com/get-your-mojo-back. Talk to your friends, your family, your other half. Join in the conversation or ask me your questions on Insta @andbreathewellbeing. I'm here for you.

How to Use This Book
The Chapters
Get Your Mojo Back is divided into seven chapters, each one covering physical, mental and practical aspects that can affect your sexual experience and relationship. Each chapter contains a personal experience that you might relate to – and, crucially, can help you understand that if you do, you're not alone. We'll cover the reasons behind these issues, and how they manifest. At the end of each chapter, you'll find tips that will put you on the right path to improve your particular situation.

Then vs Now: Exploring the History and Context of Modern Motherhood
This is mostly a book about the here and now – I want to help you with the pain and issues that impact so many of us currently. But it's also important to delve a little into how we view ourselves as women and the societal context of body image, sexuality and child-bearing. I can't do this without dissecting these cultural stereotypes, and also touching briefly on the history of sexuality and how women are viewed. I cover this in the first chapter. It's worth a read, because this background is designed to help you understand more about why you feel what you feel, and this is key to understanding the layers on top of the physical symptoms you might be experiencing.

Real-Life Stories vs Data

You've probably already guessed that I'm open about my experiences and that I think they're important for educating on a topic as sensitive as this one. But, of course, there is a lot of expert data and information that feeds into the book alongside the necessary details. There's a growing list of studies from specialists in these fields, all of which contribute to what you'll read, process and learn. I won't go heavy on the details of these references or studies in the main body text, because I want this to be a fun read (really!), so look for them at the back of the book in the bibliography if you want to find out more.

As well as weaving my own story and experiences through the book, I've included two kinds of expert voices: The Word on the Street, straight from the mouths of real-life women (and men) who are dealing with just the same shit that you are, and Get Your Mojo Back 101, to pass on words of wisdom from experts in the fields of physiotherapy/physical therapy, psychology, massage and more.

Notes on Language and Terms

Please be aware that some of the experiences I describe may be triggering if you have been through something similar yourself. If you would like further help in processing these, please contact your GP or therapist, or take a look at the resources at the back of the book.

Most of you reading will be familiar with most of the technical and medical terms I use. If you need an explanation or you're reading to support someone in your life, check out the Glossary at the back of the book.

I use terms such as postnatal and postpartum interchangeably, as well as referring with equal regularity to pelvic floor lifts and Kegels. The terms physical therapist in North American English and physiotherapist in British English refer to the same profession.

Next Steps: How to Find Out More

Each chapter features a *What Next?* section covering specific problems and how you might solve them. Read to the end of the book; there might be topics relevant to you that you weren't aware of, and in the last section you'll find chapter-specific resources including suggested further reading and lots more resources, professionals and organisations which can put you on the right path to improved intimacy.

With all the information from professionals across pregnancy, postnatal and perimenopause specialisms, plus tips and tricks to polish around the edges that you'll find in this book, *Get Your Mojo Back* might not be a magic wand, but it's a damn good start.

The whole topic of postpartum sex can sometimes be worrying and confusing, and I hope that by the end of the book you'll be feeling more enlightened and hopeful, but if you need a hand, I've put a decision tree at the end to help you find your answers. It's also important that you continue to discuss your issues openly and honestly with your other half if you have one – there are two people in this relationship!

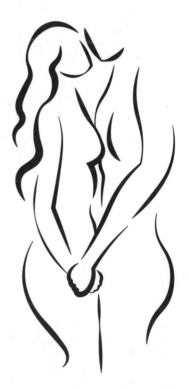

You can join the convo online @andbreathewellbeing #getyourmojoback or email clio@andbreathewellbeing. com, but of course don't hesitate to refer yourself on for further help if you need it.

Let's do it!

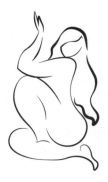

WHAT THE HELL IS OUR PROBLEM?

Why we think the way we do about sex and our bodies.

Talk honestly and openly to your buddies, and at some point you'll come on to food and/or fitness. Often this will spark conversations about weight, and perhaps clothes sizes, both of which are bound up in body image and self-confidence issues. We usually talk about ourselves in quite disparaging tones – as if there's something to improve – and though men are not immune to image-related nerves, traditionally our bodies are quite the preoccupation for women. You're probably already aware that it's a reflection of the context that surrounds us, and you might even be raging about the fact, glass of red in hand.

Bear with me, because we need to go a bit deeper into this. The historical background and the accepted norms of current society massively impact our self-image and self-worth (probably way more than they should) in ways we don't always realise. This chapter scratches the surface of the messaging that surrounds us, to nudge us just a little harder into exploring how we unintentionally interpret it, and how much that affects us. Spoiler alert: quite a lot, actually.

It's important to start here because both pregnancy and childbirth are acts of the body as well as of sex. Your body changes: it grows, shrinks, earns stripes and functions vastly differently than before. You're a multi-faceted goddess, with magical abilities to create life, but navigating these chameleon stages in relatively quick succession can also be a bit of a head-fuck.

You start with an already-confused view of yourself and your sexuality, and move into an even more bewildering whirlwind of perspectives and feelings. And hormones; let's not forget hormones.

I think that to understand the impact of pregnancy and childbirth on sex and relationships in the postnatal period, parenthood and later in life, we need to start with some historical perspective and an exploration of cultural norms. Plus, this will give you more ammo for those dinner party conversations.

A Potted History of Sexuality

Let's pause and rewind. Historically – or make that *her*storically – pleasure had a very small role to play in the female experience of sex. Women engaged passively with intercourse, seeing it as something to be endured rather than enjoyed (even now we're familiar with the phrase ". . . lie back and think of England").[1] And who can blame us, when women in the past spent most of their adult lives pregnant or preparing to conceive, and becoming an adult meant sexual maturity at a far younger age than now – Shakespeare's Juliet was only 13 years old, and we consider her one half of the greatest romantic couple in English Literature. Women were expected to have babies one after the other, and those with fertility issues were considered failures.

I'm sure there were exceptions; however, during most historical periods, contemporary evidence suggests that hopping into bed with your husband was usually some way down the list of fun Saturday-night activities.[2] Sex was for procreating, not creating pleasure. Plus we bore the brunt of all the child-rearing in between pregnancies.

For example, in Renaissance Europe, the average woman could expect to give birth up to seven times in a life span of under 40 years, or up to ten times if she was lucky enough to live to 45 years old.[3] Suffice to say, the amount of time between pregnancies was short. Breastfeeding acts as the body's natural defence by delaying your next pregnancy (your menstrual cycle is not likely to return to normal until after you stop the boob), so if you used a wet nurse, the respite period would be even shorter.

Even worse, your babies might not even survive. *You* might not survive. Here's a stark fact: childbirth was so dangerous that until fairly recently, most wealthy women would make their wills on becoming pregnant – it's fair to say it was no picnic. And with vintage contraception ineffective, and frankly, at times disgusting (mouse poo or pigeon droppings were ingredients in two delightful ancient Roman suggestions[4]), women's sexual pleasure was some way down the list of priorities.

Consider this: while in Roman times orgies were common, women were usually not the focus. For example, you might already know that it was common for men to take adolescent boys as companions (though there's still debate over how much sex went on in these homosexual couplings) and that women were relegated to the role of child-bearing vessels.

So, because sex would ideally lead to pregnancy, and because infant survival rates were low and life expectancies short, not being ready for sex postnatally just wasn't an option. In fact, women have spent a lot of history as the property of men – the legal concept of coverture (when a woman becomes subsumed under a man's identity in marriage) existed in Britain until the late 19th century,[5] and when something is viewed as property rather than a person, feelings are rendered irrelevant. See white people's abhorrent treatment of black slaves as a case in point.

Female slaves were routinely raped and made pregnant by white masters and overseers, as well as other slaves. This heritage and historical trauma doesn't leave you without a little baggage echoing down the generations. The detail of this topic is not mine to tell, so the Bibliography at the back of this book has some brilliant further reading for you if you want to learn more about race and sexuality.

I'm rounding up this whistle-stop tour with a word on religion, because the often-violent global spread of Christianity meant that sex came to be viewed as dirty, and not in a nudge-nudge, wink-wink kinda way. More in a hellfire and brimstone kinda way.[6] Christianity is not the only faith to affect our societal views on sexuality, and arguably religious prudishness has had the longest-lasting impact on our current societal expectations.

The Victorians nicely illustrate my point about the sway of Christianity: they were particularly good at promoting an awful dichotomy between chaste marriages – "good" women only do it once a month, please – against the background of abundant, usually working-class, prostitution. This predictably resulted in a sexual underworld and thence widespread venereal disease, which even the most "proper" families didn't escape: did you know that Churchill's dad, Lord Randolph, had syphilis?[7] This historical tradition has clear parallels with today's tension between pressure to have sex and slut-shaming – about which I talk more in this chapter.

While we find ourselves a long way in time from these chronicled women, I think most of you will find, as I do, that the tensions between our bodies, our sexuality, the pressure to be "good", childbirth and the fine line between pleasure and pain are close and relatable. My own story illustrates a journey that I know most, if not all of you, will empathise with. I know this because I've spoken about it a lot, and always received relieved and tearful responses. So my passion, pun intended, for this topic stems from there.

I'm not saying that great sex is the be-all and end-all of a partnership, but it's a bloody good start. *Your* journey from painful, emotionally taxing intimacy back to enjoyable sex and a fulfilling relationship is one that's important too. We might not talk openly about sex (at least not with a straight face – bad jokes don't count), but it's at the heart of your marriage/partnership and the basis of a happy relationship. And a happy relationship = a happy family.

Why all the jokes? Why the hiding? We don't take our own sex lives seriously because we're embarrassed and we don't think we're worth the time. To uncover more, I'll build on the brief historical context above to further explain about the current societal context around our identity as women and as mothers. To be clear, dads and other partner parents are important in this journey too, and we'll explore the male perspective and input from fathers and partners later in the book, but the huge physical and mental changes wrought through pregnancy and childbirth fall to women. For now, at least.

So here I am, giving you a window into my own journey – from uncertain self-image through pregnancy and birth – and how it affected me. I want you to know that all births are okay: there is no perfect birth, just the birth you experienced. Whatever that birth looks like – joyful and water-based or elective caesarean or traumatic – it will probably impact you physically and mentally in a positive or negative way, or probably a bit of both. I'll also talk in more depth about birth trauma later in the book.

My Story

I hated my body growing up. I am short, still only 5'1", but my breasts budded early and I became softer, rounder, while my friends were becoming taller and ganglier. I read teen magazines stuffed with models and watched traditionally beautiful actors on TV, and I absorbed the message that my body wasn't good enough. Even though the body I had was good at sport, acted in lead roles, played three musical instruments and had a smart brain, those things didn't register as important. I didn't look how others did and I was convinced I wasn't good enough. The fact that I didn't have queues of boyfriends as a teenager underlined to me that I wasn't worthy. I loved and despised food in equal measure. My inner critic grew strong.

In the summer before university, I lost my puppy fat and found my healthy weight, and with it a new and unexpected confidence. I now perceived I was better looking, and therefore was now worth seeing and making time for. I felt deserving of the new wave of approbation from boys.

Now I'd had a taste of adulation, I'd have done anything to keep it. Having not had many boyfriends at school, at university I discovered I was popular. My eating became disordered, and I hooked up with a lot of people. My self-worth was intrinsically tied to what I ate and who I slept with. I developed an unhealthy relationship with food and men, and all because I thought I was going to feel better about myself.

I see now that I was goaded too. We all acted like that, laughing about the number of conquests, being admired, adored, but also judged for it. We felt we had to drink and be one of the gang, but woe betide us if the partying meant we put on weight. We awarded ourselves bragging rights over men, but simultaneously found ourselves whispered about when we had behaved "like a whore". What a fine line to walk. We were judged by men but we judged ourselves more harshly. There is nothing like the bitchiness of women, egged on by men.

In my twenties I edged my way toward self-compassion. It was the start of the path to where I am now, but it still took that entire decade to find peace with myself. I discovered how to balance eating well and having fun, and how not to judge myself against impossible standards. I found routine in my fitness, getting stronger and functionally fit rather than trying to lose weight. I discovered a man who could support me emotionally and argue with me healthily, who valued me and wanted to be with me because I was me, not because I was promiscuous or suitably thin.

After the early relationship ups and downs, three years after we met, we got married. A couple of years after that we decided to try for a baby, and that's when all the things that I thought I had conquered came back for round two. The balance I had achieved was positioned on a knife edge and required constant monitoring and a thought-through routine to maintain it. We talked about having a baby, but I'd never been broody or considered myself very maternal. It seemed like something we wanted to do, to create a life together, but I wasn't desperate for a baby. Added to which I was fearful and uncertain about how I would cope with the changes in my body.

Nearing my thirties, I was finally in a position to accept my body, with a balanced exercise routine, an honest relationship with food and contentment with my self-image. But getting pregnant and pushing a baby out, and the changes in my body that would go with it, would surely challenge that. I was scared of ballooning. I was scared of not being able to exercise. I was scared of not being able to control what I was eating. I was scared of stretch marks. I was scared of not "getting my body back" postnatally. And I was petrified of the birth: the pain, the scarring, the damage to my pelvic floor.

My self-acceptance was based on being in charge of my own destiny. Pregnancy and childbirth are not big on letting you control your own body. You can't predict how you're going to feel in pregnancy, or how your body will cope. Whether your mind will get itself into a spin or be completely zen. You just don't know what factors might impact your birth, or whether you'll be lucky or unlucky. So despite having agreed to get pregnant and being happy with the decision, the unknown factors and lack of control left me see-sawing over the prospect of becoming a mother. I would be excited about having a little being of my own in my arms, and then, via nerves over my body's ability to recover and how I would be judged, go careering down a birth-horror-story rabbit hole in my mind. Only looking back on it do I recognise that I probably had mild birth fear, which in its severest form is recognised as tokophobia. It was all far from ideal.

Almost as if my body knew I was wary, I became pregnant quickly. I was lucky to come off the pill and get pregnant very soon afterwards. I didn't have a post-pill period, so I didn't realise I was pregnant until a month or two later, when my bleed still hadn't arrived. I had assumed it might take some time, perhaps up to a year, to try for a baby successfully, so my mind hadn't fully adjusted to the idea of being pregnant. When I finally thought to do a pregnancy test, I felt selfish for crying when it was positive.

I didn't know it, but by the time I took that pregnancy test I was about eight weeks pregnant. It's amazing how something so momentous can happen without you even realising it. I took the test around Christmas time, so with holiday closures and waiting times, it wasn't until the New Year that I managed to get my first midwife appointment at the hospital. I was three months gone without even knowing it. Because I had had little time to adjust and it felt to me (though it wasn't) unplanned, I ignored my pregnancy, carrying on as normal. I was competent, confident, independent. Nothing to see here!

I hated losing control of my body, which I'd worked so hard to come to terms with through my twenties, and I felt nauseated for the whole nine-plus months, all day every day. Playing down the pregnancy meant that I also swept the prospect of the birth under the carpet. Despite being engaged in the usual antenatal classes, perhaps I didn't really imagine the birth was going to happen (or hoped it wasn't). Who looks forward to the image of birth that we're schooled on? The screaming, sweating women in pain on television and in films?

Being a Lover, a Mother and Everything Else

There's a cartoon doing the rounds; you've probably seen it. It's by the amazing French illustrator, Emma, and it's called "You Should've Asked".[8] Emma's work explores the heartbreaking cultural acceptance of the (often unacknowledged) female workload in the household, which regularly comes on top of the child-rearing burden and in addition to a job or career outside of the home. This unacknowledged work is often called the "mental load" and consists of anything and everything, from the weekly grocery shop, tax and insurance admin, buying presents and remembering birthdays, to organising family events, booking holidays and cleaning.

I mention it here, because it's an important illustration of the conflict that resides within all women. The fight to stand on our own two feet and be recognised as equal has meant that our ability in work, politics and sporting and cultural endeavours has grown, but at the same time the household burden has rarely shifted. That means that in most families, we still get to do all that other shit. No biggie.

Whether you think we're complicit in this situation by not fighting hard enough against it or you don't (and I don't, by the way), the fact is we usually occupy multiple different identities at once. The professional woman or worker or earner, the homemaker, the sister, the daughter . . . and the lover. When you throw "mother" into the mix, is it any wonder our heads are in a spin?

It's hard enough to be clear on what you want from one of these roles or how you choose to personify it, let alone fulfilling them all. What happens when you transition between two of them, or two seemingly opposing identities vie for attention at the same time?

We're going to focus on two of these attention-seekers (obviously my faves): the Lover and the Mother. On the surface, we usually jump into the family game without much thought; but I know that in reality there is far more going on in those little heads of ours – these days there are even therapists specialising in helping women decide whether or not to have children. Unpack what both Lover and Mother mean to you, and lots of further questions arise.

If you think of your role as Lover, for example, you might consider the following:

- When did you become sexually active?
- How physically developed were you at the time?
- How did you feel about your body?
- Were you emotionally ready?
- Was it a loving and intimate experience?
- Did you feel pressured into sex?
- What was the dialogue among your peers about sex?
- How did your school deal with sex education?
- What has been your relationship with your own sexuality since then?

The following questions might crop up when you consider the Mother part of your identity:

- What was your relationship like with your own parents?
- Did you actively choose to become a parent or not?
- Are you still in a relationship with the baby's father?

- How loving and positive is that relationship?
- Did you enjoy being pregnant?
- Are you instinctively maternal?
- Are you taking a break from your career outside the home?
- How are you finding motherhood?

And then there's the relationship between the two:

- How easy was it to become pregnant?
- Has your body changed through pregnancy and childbirth?
- How do you feel about your body now?
- How traumatic was your birth?
- Is there a lasting physical impact?
- Are you still in pain?
- Are you affected mentally by childbirth and motherhood?
- How is your relationship with your other half?

Feel free to be a smartypants and write down some of your thoughts on a spare sheet of paper or your journal, or just scribble them in the margins here. I want this book to be helpful to you, so you can use it in whatever way you feel comfortable. Once you have thought about your answers, guess what? Whatever they are, they're bound to have been influenced by societal expectations.

Being a Lover

Most of our upbringing is shaped by the expectation of finding a partner. Jane Austen's novels are considered classics, not just because of dripping Mr Darcy, but because there's something about her subject matter that endures. While we can't all stumble upon a hot lover emerging soaking wet from a lake, we probably spent most of our teen years, and even more likely our twenties and thirties, plotting how to win one over.

We usually realise as we grow older that the more we value ourselves and the more self-confidence we have, the more attractive we are to our potential other halves. But before we get there, we spend a lot of time and money shoe-horning ourselves into the images we think they want to see. This manifests itself in the way we dress and the clothes we choose, the fashions we're told we should be following in magazines and on TV; the style of our hair, from school hairdos fussed over in the bathrooms to the subtle shame we feel over the appearance of grey hair or the frizziness that appears in humid conditions; the make-up that we paint on our faces whether we're going for siren or, ugh, "natural"; the way we hold our breath walking the fine line between sexy and not too sexy for a party so we're not slut-shamed.

It's not as simple as boys setting the rules and girls conforming, I know. There are huge pressures on boys and men, from sexual expectations to body image to the conversation around sensitivity and strength. But the framework is created by a society and history dominated by the people in charge (who are men) and perpetuated by the cultural juggernaut (whose decision-makers were also traditionally men), so that if you don't conform, if you dare to be different, you don't fit in. I truly admire those who don't care about not fitting in, but most of us feel at least mildly swayed or mentally impacted by it.

The dialogue often reads like this: you're supposed to dress and behave sexily to attract a mate. But the minute you go too far, you're a whore. We grow up and realise that this isn't fair or nice (can I get an understatement award, please?), but the impact of that start in life is like an earworm that just won't get out of your head. In other words, it's further-reaching than we think. We absorb this rhetoric and find ourselves judging others (let's face it, usually other women) subconsciously by these standards despite our badass-feminist selves.

How on earth are we supposed to manage that opposition? How are we supposed to be sexy and pure at the same time? How do we manage the guilt over hard-to-recognise subconscious bias? It's true that we inhabit many personalities at the same time – for example, we behave differently with friends than we do with family – but the Madonna–whore juxtaposition is a particularly spiteful and contrasting pairing, despite the persistence of the sexy nun Halloween costume. Yes, really.

The Word on the Street

Christina Pickworth, 40, talent agent, business owner, mum of two @thismamadoes

"Personally, I do struggle with how I feel about my body. How I feel about what it looks like. But on the other side of that, I refuse to let that be the narrative that I want to listen to. Even if I feel it, I just think, bollocks to that! I don't want to lean into that. I try to be very positive about my body now, certainly on Instagram and, you know, sometimes in real life too (!). Do I like my 40-year-old body as much as I liked my 24-year-old body? No. Am I grateful for it? Yes, enormously and that's something that I feel I can celebrate.

I think the thing that I'll always go back to is that feeling sexy doesn't come from what I look like, it comes from an inside place. So actually, if I can find the sexy, then everything else just matters a bit less. I know from things that I've read, or from talking with friends, that a lot of people just don't feel that, and that is such a shame because I do think there's this overwhelming narrative that mothers can't feel sexy. You end up suppressing it, I think, either within a relationship or perhaps because there's such a lot of narrative about shame or guilt around sex and how women are supposed to behave. And so much [narrative] about women being or not being sexual . . . and often being called promiscuous. And so I think depending on what your experience has been, perhaps you could shut that bit down. For me it's like a flame really deep inside and something that I think is probably quite easy to bury.

When people talk about depression and anxiety, often there's talk about how that might limit libido. For me, it probably goes the other way, but probably in an unhealthy way. Because I think, for me, it was a way to feel something. Not at the moment, but with hindsight, in earlier periods of my life, I can see that perhaps that's how I used it.

Some other narratives of sexuality and motherhood feel to me to be telling a story that's opposite to my experience. There's a lot of 'it's okay to be tired' and 'it's okay to not fancy [sex]'. Whereas for me, I always felt like I was at the opposite end of the spectrum: 'I'm still here!' I want to be the person that is ringing the bell for still getting jiggy with it! It's okay if you don't! But lots of us are still really up for it: it can feel quite lonely, like 'Is no one having sex?! What's wrong with me then?'

It's so tiring that the [narrative] that's offered up is one or the other. We need to hear more stories; in the same way that motherhood is every shade of grey, sex drive and sexuality are every shade of grey too. And I do think part of that is this idea that men have a high sex drive and women don't enjoy sex, or all men enjoy sex more than women. Which is nonsense and exacerbates it all."

Being a Mother

And what about being a mother? The archetypal homely, apron-wearing, baking woman in the kitchen might be a 1950s wet dream, rather than a 2020s fantasy, but there's an element of relevance still. As well as implying frumpiness, the idea of motherhood lacks glamour, featuring a focus on child-rearing and home-making, and the expectation that all of this is kept in hand in addition to any other activities (like, say, a career). The stereotype of motherhood contains a woman neatly in a box, within boundaries that control and keep her, and it's a very different stereotype to that of the Lover.

Ultimately, the Mother is a de-sexualised persona. There's a reason the MILF and the Cougar are such fetishised versions of women. The MILF ("Mother I'd like to fuck", in case you didn't know) is a taboo figure. Mothers are not meant to be sexy, so when they are, it's perceived as illicit. The MILF is a refinement of the Cougar – an older woman with a younger lover, uncompromising in her sexuality – again an illicit juxtaposition of age and/or motherhood with passion. But it's precisely the act of being a lover which leads to motherhood. We can't win!

For most of us, it's a fine line to tread, balancing these two ideas and finding our place within each of these identities, and that's totally normal. It's an odd situation in which we are expected to go seamlessly from one to the other, and it's not surprising that this might prove difficult for some. It did for me. And if it does for you, you're not alone.

Assessing your identity as a new mother is hard enough without the added weight of losing your old identity and all the ramifications that has on your sexuality (itself a large piece of the identity puzzle). We usually find that when we become mothers, we step from a place of confidence and self-assuredness into the unknown. With a lack of support network and education around the postnatal period, we often question our own knowledge, physical ability (difficulty breastfeeding, slow healing, all the crying – yours as well as the baby's!) and intuition (though we often know best). Where the fuck is that child-raising village I was promised? It's only natural that we question ourselves over everything.

So, going against the grain of expectation, how do we rediscover our strength, our confidence and our sexuality, so that we (and our partners) are once more happy and satisfied? Lack of confidence isn't sexy, so besides the very real issues of physical and mental healing, identity plays a bigger role than we realise in the happiness of our relationships. It's hard to quantify, and therefore often hard to recognise. I'm here to help you do that.

The Word on the Street

Natalie Lee, 42, author of *Feeling Myself*, speaker, mum of two @stylemesunday

"How I feel about my body has been a huge rollercoaster. I think the most significant change happened after I had children. I suddenly had a very different perspective on my body, I really struggled with how it looked after childbirth. During pregnancy, I actually felt my most sexy and most embodied. Because I could take pictures and I wasn't sucking in my stomach, I was actually proud to have this big stomach for the first time ever. I felt very womanly, like my body was doing its job.

And then afterwards, I was left with a saggy stomach; I was left with stretch marks that all came in the last week of pregnancy when I went overdue. I had all this water retention. I felt like my body had been run over by a truck and put back together again. I also didn't realise until later that I was dealing with issues of feeling that my body had let me down, because I ended up having an emergency caesarean. I didn't realise how much of that had impacted my view of my body and my self-esteem.

Working through that was a very long, slow process of realisations, [. . .] lightbulb moments. I didn't realise that I had internalised the notion that my body had let me down. [But when I did,] I had to sit down and really mourn that thought process. It was good: that awareness was a really important moment for me. That sparked this desire to change my mentality about my body. I realised how shit I felt about my body, and having children; it just gives you this other perspective. I started to question and challenge these notions I had [about my body] and where they were coming from. Because suddenly I was seeing it through the eyes of my children, and I thought, I don't want them to grow up not questioning things, thinking that their bodies are not their own, thinking that their bodies are for the consumption of other people and that they are intrinsically never good enough!

I always felt nothing was ever good enough. No matter how slim I was, no matter how smooth my skin was, no matter how much attention I got from other people. So I worked really hard on questioning my beliefs about my body. I started to explore my own body, whereas I hadn't really before: I learned about my body through the exploration of other people's hands rather than my own. So actually, I really found my sexiness in my thirties – as a mother. I started to explore myself and masturbate, and I just started to feel more at home in my body because I was challenging a lot of these inbuilt notions that I wasn't even aware of before.

There's a serious lack of desire to educate women about female pleasure and feeling at home in your body. I realised only after I had children that I'd never thought that my body was my own. The only thing I was interested in (in terms of how I looked and whether I was sexy) was whether it was attractive to other people. I saw myself through the eyes of other people, never through my own eyes.

For me it was also about race, about hair. I didn't look like the women in the magazines that I read – I was really into *Just Seventeen* and *Jackie*, and I didn't see a representation of me in those magazines. And that hugely affected my identity and my ability to think that I was beautiful. I was brought up by a mum who was white and I didn't have much connection to the black side of my family. So the whole of my childhood I wanted to be white. I wanted to have long flowy blonde hair that you're able to flick around when you're in bed!

When I was younger, I would have separated my identity from my sexuality. Now I feel like my sexuality is an intrinsic part of who I am, and I am very, very aware of controlling the narrative around my own sexuality.

The way we view and categorise women is so one-dimensional. You're either this or that. No, I'm all of them. I speak to my children about female sexuality, pleasure and why have we demonised it, why we are silencing it. That stuff only perpetuates the shame aspect that we link to female sexuality.

After I had children, I felt like I lost my identity because you're so wrapped up in nappies. It was almost like starting from the bottom: 'Who am I now? Who the fuck am I?' That took a long time. That 'me', she's still here. And she's also not there. And she's also a sexual person. There's a lot of judgement from other people on who we should be now as mothers. It is really difficult to disengage with that judgement and rediscover your own personal values and identity. We underestimate how difficult that is.

Motherhood is romanticised so extremely. I wanted to be a mother for a very long time before I was one. I was desperate, absolutely desperate. And I felt like I was going to be a very holistic organic [mother], at one with my child. Nothing else mattered. The reality was absolutely nothing like the vision that I had. And that's the issue. We're not talking about the reality of motherhood. We don't warn people about how it strips your whole identity and how difficult it is. I really struggled with feeling like I had been lied to my whole life. Because no one warned me. And that's not fucking fair.

How I feel about my body has had, and does have, a massive impact on my sexual side. The main issue is the ability to be present. If I'm not feeling good about my body, I can't be present in terms of being a sexual person. And therefore I'm not able to enjoy myself. The two are inextricably linked. As my confidence and self-esteem increase, so does my sexual pleasure and desire."

The Twilight Zone

When you become pregnant, you inhabit a twilight zone between Lover and Mother. You're a mother without a child. A lover without the sexiness. Though you can't have one without the other, depending on your journey to pregnancy, the relationship between these two identities might be fraught.

Pregnancy causes the body to change, and our body image and self-confidence can be altered. For many of us with fraught, complicated or simply "normal" relationships with our bodies, pregnancy adds another layer of stress to that relationship. No wonder, then, that sex might become an unwitting victim of pregnancy. While some of us are high on hormones and find ourselves super-horny during pregnancy, others find that we shy away from intimacy, embarrassed about our changing bodies, or are simply not used to the practical physical difficulties of sex with an enormous bump, already-tender boobs, fatigue or nausea.

If the road to pregnancy has been a long one, your body may seem to have let you down, and it's hard to cultivate a loving relationship with your other half when you don't have one with your own body. Mentally, the conflict between sex as a pleasurable and intimate part of your relationship and sex as a necessary chore in order to start a family is a common one for IVF or adoption couples that drives away joy and breeds resentment.

If you aren't sure whether you want to have a baby or not, but have started trying for the first time, or if you're on your second time around and you're not sure you're ready, you may be holding back during sex.

So even before you're postnatal, you're building the foundations for your sex life post-baby. That could be positive, but more often than not it's neutral or even negative. Whatever it is, that's okay. If it's negative, it doesn't have to be permanent. Just being aware is the first step toward a happier bedtime.

The Damned Patriarchy

It's an oldie but a goodie, and doesn't it keep rearing its ugly head? In all but the rarest examples, societies are dominated and framed by men. Matriarchal societies are few and far between – the Mosuo is a fascinating and rare example in China, near the border with Tibet.[9] So in the rest of the world, we are left with a framework created largely by men, and this is usually the lens through which we view ourselves in society – divided into men, women and children. But what the hell does that mean?

It means that because of the bias throughout history toward male dominance in property and land ownership, jobs, politics, wealth and more, male opinions and values are those that matter the most in society and the ones by which we tend to live. Those with the power make the rules. And despite making steps toward equality over the last century in particular (slow and steady wins the race, eh?), values take much longer to shift, especially if they are subconsciously held.

Most of the women I speak to are feminists, and most of the men too, even if they don't call themselves that. This conversation is not necessarily about feminism or the archetypal bra-burning feminist: feminists can still 100 per cent wear pink, and I strongly feel you can inhabit whatever personality you like and still be a feminist. But it's still rare to come across a person who is not defined, at least in part, by the gender in which they were raised, whether they identify as feminist or not.

Moving Back or Moving Forward? Why Language Matters

It might not surprise you to learn that I don't like the terms "bouncing back", "back into shape" or "got her body back". I think they're supremely unhelpful. Firstly, where the hell do you think it's gone? It's always been here and it's okay for it to change shape. Secondly, growing an actual human being inside your own body is an incredible feat, and if the souvenirs of that astonishing journey are visible, then that's alright by me.

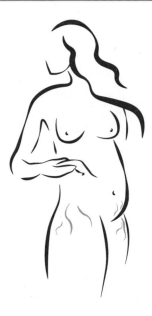

Thirdly, men seem to age and grow their paunches with a remarkable lack of comment (sometimes with a bit of fetishisation actually – "dad-bod", anyone?), so why should we be subjected to it?

I've tried to be positive about the message I'm sending in this book, because I believe we need all the support we can get through this postnatal and motherhood journey, and that changing our internal dialogue is sometimes easier said than done. So although this book, and hopefully all the wonderful people you choose to read, watch and follow on social media are shouting to you about yourself and your post-birth body in a positive way, I think this lesson is about more than what you consume. It's about how that manifests in your mind too.

What I mean is, yes, you can read this stuff and know intellectually that you don't need to bounce back, that you're marvellous just as you are. But when it comes to how you subconsciously react, how you secretly feel about yourself and your body, it can often be a different story. If you can embed that knowledge by talking about it, applying it to yourself, saying it out loud in the mirror (you know I love a good affirmation), you'll be even more of a rock star than you are already.

I'm not saying that you have to be totally in love with your body (but if you are, that's brilliant); accepting it and acknowledging the work it's done is enough. We're not bouncing back, we're moving forward into this new body of ours (whether that looks like the same body you had before or not) and into this new identity. Stop yearning for where you were. The body you have now is the one you'll be looking back on with regret in ten years' time. Time moves forward, and we move forward. Your postnatal recovery and your body in motherhood is not about going backward, or about trying to retrieve something you've lost. It's about embracing its journey onward and cherishing what you've gained. So there.

More of the Damned Patriarchy?

From these gender characteristics, society develops stereotypes of both men and women. Stereotypes can be helpful to understand how to view others, but more often they can restrict the way that we view ourselves and also the way we operate in life. For women, this can most often shape the way that we think about ourselves and our body image. In the fragile teen years, it's easy to reflect back others' opinions of how you "should" look and dress, and it's usually this adolescent period that most quickly shapes our view of ourselves and our confidence.

Two identities at opposing ends of the spectrum that get a lot of airtime are the Siren and the Mother. The Siren, or the sex symbol, is the embodiment of the female goal of attracting a mate, the view of women purely in relation to men, the act of defining the female appearance via the male gaze. And the Mother is the "ultimate" – biological – purpose of the child-bearing woman, the achievement of the goal of nurturing and giving care to both her children and her partner. Most women inhabit (more or less) both of these two personalities over the course of their lives, as well as plenty of others. Let's give ourselves a pat on the back for our chameleon achievements, as at the heart of this switcheroo is the moment you have a baby.

As well as the male gaze framework (that old chestnut), let's not forget the smaller framework in which we're raised – our family. We've probably all heard Philip Larkin's poem "This Be The Verse".[10] You might not recognise the title, but I bet you know at least the opening lines about your parents fucking you up – Google them, because I'm not supposed to print any more of it here. And I think good old Philip was right on the money in some ways. More recently, his namesake Philippa Perry has dived deeply and eloquently into the subject of parental behaviour being passed on to our children and how to lessen the impact of negative traits on our next generation.[11] And there's no shortage of parenting literature in between.

In a nutshell, children are emotional and behavioural sponges. Our childhood family environment, the views, the rules, the emotional relationship, the examples of our parents all contribute to how we view ourselves. So – klaxon alert! – the way that your mum thought about her body and the way that she viewed herself as a mother, in her career, as a lover (whether this was verbally expressed or not) will all impact how you view yourself in exactly those situations.

You probably don't think of your parents, particularly your mother, as sexual beings. Even we are victims of historical patterns, and this is why it's especially hard to fit our new prenatal and postnatal identities together with our existing ones..

What I'm saying is that the role of women in society – sorry to get heavy, but this stuff is important – has a big impact on how you feel about yourself after you have a baby. New motherhood can be a completely mind-bending time in more ways than one. But you're not alone, and (let's break out the therapist talk) this situation is often shaped by things that are out of your control. In other words: it might not be your fault, but you can do something about it.

Get Your Mojo Back 101

Sarah Forbes – anthropologist, sexual culturalist and author @mamasexbook

"It wasn't until I became an adult that I realised that I was raised in a very unique environment when it came to the body and how I should think about my body and self-confidence. I actually think it was because my own mother had many issues with those topics. But she never pushed those on me. She never talked about what I ate or commented on my body. Instead, she made me look in the mirror and say 'I am Sarah. I am confident.'

A lot of us, as mothers, are saying we want to fix various cycles that have flourished in our families and society. We want to promote body positivity in our homes, we want our children to feel comfortable in their bodies in general, but also with their sexual expression and identity when that becomes age appropriate. There's this energy of wanting to fix wrongs for our children, even if we don't necessarily know how to fix them for ourselves.

When it comes to sex and body education, there is a big gap in conscious parenting (potentially wanting to do it in a different way than our parents) and addressing for ourselves how we were raised to think about these topics, and how we engage in our own education now as adults. We were supposed to have learned these things long ago, when we were much younger, not after becoming a mother. But in actuality, motherhood is a unique opportunity because you become a new person (with, in some ways, a new body), and getting to know that person is a critical, exciting and profound opportunity.

There's a shocking deficit in our education on *matrescence*, or the mom version of adolescence. The identity shift [to motherhood] can be quite painful because we're not prepared for it. If you knew it was coming, you wouldn't be so shocked when you went through that chapter. In hindsight, it's obvious. Your body has done this hugely transformative thing, your social role is completely changed. We've finally come to this place where we can own our pregnant body publicly in a way that we couldn't in previous eras, but we struggle to own the shift in our person into motherhood, primarily because we lack education on it.

I'm using social media as my ethnographic fieldwork for my book *Mama Sex*, as it allows me to study the different tribes of mothers or the different cultures of motherhood. In some ways the self-created images and expectations of real mothers are so much more powerful than what we're receiving from magazines and other media representations. Within motherhood, if you're struggling or having any kind of challenge, the question always arises: 'Am I a good mother?' Society has created that anxiety and fear in us, rooted in the 'perfect mother myth' to keep us on the hamster wheel, one that gets perpetuated on social media.

Historically, we've said a sexual mother is a bad mother. The trap of all of this is that if you do anything that is about you, your own pleasure, your own autonomy, society slaps you with the 'bad mother' label. If you are scared you're going to be judged for [taking back that power], it comes back to the pervasiveness of the 'perfect mother' myth. We self-police: we learn that motherhood is about prioritising others, and what could be more selfish than pleasure?

Before you had children, you probably allowed yourself a diversity and fluidity of sexual expression, whereas in motherhood almost any expression [of sexuality] kicks you into whore versus Madonna territory. When we enter motherhood, any energy around our sexuality is intensified, because of long-held taboos on the topic. With my book I'm teasing out many different histories: the history of motherhood, what we expect of mothers, but also the history of female sexuality, which, for thousands of years, has been about *controlling* female sexuality. Hammurabi's Code [an ancient Mesopotamian text inscribed around 1792–1750 BCE] is all about restricting women's sexuality: women and children were property. If a woman is having sex with whomever she wants, that property line isn't secure. But if you control her sexuality and reproduction, you're controlling everything. In a way, we're asking society to undo, in the 50 or 60 years since the sexual revolution, thousands of years of precedent.

I'm seeing a modern motherhood revolution: it's in our own homes, with our bodies, as well as with what we're doing to reclaim ourselves as individuals. It really is historically revolutionary. People say it's so hard to change the patriarchy, but we do have micro-abilities to enact change: our own sexuality is one of them. I can claim even the tiniest space and it's totally mine – the system isn't going to come and police my orgasm!

Our brains, not our bodies, are the centres of our erotic selves. We all have different erotic blueprints and we have to give ourselves permission to explore (while fantasy and thoughts are the driver of sexuality for some, for others touch and sensation are a tremendous part of the sexual experience). We assume that we know everything about ourselves, rather than being open to getting to know 'new' versions, which is essential in the pregnancy, postpartum and motherhood shift. It's about continuing to explore; we should always be evolving and changing. No body, no one, no identity and no relationship is stagnant.

We need to keep this in mind with age and ageing (which is perceived as a negative because society has constructed it in this way). A lot of mothers are having children later in life, going through all the changes of motherhood and then slamming into perimenopausal waters or menopause. This makes it so hard to know the true origin of our physical shifts or identity-changing needs. Are these changes that would be occurring even if you weren't a mother? That's something to think about."

What Next?

Alright, so what do we do about all of this? Here's the good stuff.

- Think about the view you have of yourself both physically and mentally, and whether it's changed since having a baby.
- Recognise that it's a hard transition to make to go from one stereotype to another, crossing a wide gulf to do so.
- Pinpoint any differences in your identity and know that whatever you're feeling, it's normal, and that usually we are impacted disproportionately by the societal framework we're brought up in.
- Talk to your other half about how you are feeling. Sometimes men, or non-birthing partners, don't understand the impact of cultural expectations. Talk to your friends too – if you open up, the chances are they are going (or have been) through something similar.
- Visit your GP if you are feeling low. The baby blues are extremely common and expected, as hormones fluctuate after birth, but if it lasts longer, reach out for help. This includes experiencing negative emotions toward sex, your partner or your baby, feeling large amounts of anxiety, rage, depression or experiencing psychosis. There are more signposts in Chapter 2 and at the back of this book.

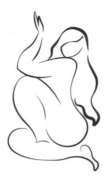

SO WHAT EXACTLY AM I DEALING WITH?

Unpicking the changes in your body, hormones, identity and mental health.

In among all the nappy-buying, moving to a bigger home, fitting in antenatal classes and fending off the strangers' hands trying to feel your bump, there's surprisingly little time to come to terms with becoming a mother. We assume that things will somehow carry on as normal, or prepare ourselves and worry about the things we *think* will change, which often are not the things that *actually* will. Instead, there's a whole other set of things we need to practise.

In this chapter I want to look at how this lack of understanding of the changes in our bodies and lifestyle (or is it a refusal to acknowledge them?), plus the associated fear of the changes we *are* aware of, impacts our bodies and our minds.

A beautiful set of pictures by Natasha Sena[1] points out some of the things we should have been training for instead of birth: the wake-ups ("Set an alarm for every two hours."), the fact that you just can't leave the house without forgetting at least three things and being at least 20 minutes behind schedule

("Say you're leaving. Then don't. Repeat."), the weird feeling of attachment even when they're not on you ("Fall asleep sitting down then wake up screaming: where is the baby?") and the fact that often it's all on you, and you might feel more in tune with the baby than your other half ("Wake up only to watch your husband sleep peacefully.")

Because not only does a baby come into your life, though that's monumental enough, but your life shifts completely too. That means physically, mentally, emotionally and sexually.

Why do we not talk about the changes we go through? Why is it such a secret that we might experience incontinence? That the first postpartum poo is hideous? That we might have scarring and aches that we weren't prepared for and don't know how to fix? In some senses, though we're often looking for ways to get back to the person we were before motherhood, we might never get there. That doesn't have to be a bad thing, but it does require some preparation and adjustment. We should be forewarned, and we rarely are.

I used to think this secrecy was about hiding how bad childbirth can be, and the desperate sleepless nights of new parenthood. That this secrecy was shrouding the truth so that women wouldn't be put off starting a family. It often feels like it might be a kind of sisterhood secret – for women particularly, not men, as traditionally their lives change relatively little. Like if we knew how painful birth could be, or how we might nearly lose our minds with fatigue, we would be less likely to bear children.

Or perhaps the evasion of these truths is less deliberate, and more of a collective memory loss, brought on by the coo of a contented baby (which can be as rare as hen's teeth). Those gummy smiles are magical things. Either way, it was worth it in the end. Hopefully.

I might argue that underlying this secrecy is the cultural acceptance that the difficulties and changes brought about by childbirth are inherently a female problem, a symptom of our entrenched patriarchal system. This makes it a sort of wilful ignorance of how hard pregnancy, birth and motherhood can be. And then we perpetuate it by not talking about it (the sisterhood secret) . . . does that mean we're complicit in our own entrapment? Eek, that's a scary thought.

Whatever the reason, it means that we're often woefully underprepared for motherhood. Our expectations are skewed. The timelines of where we think our bodies and minds and sex lives should be are completely out of whack with the wobbly reality of new, and not-so-new, motherhood.

This means that mentally, physically and sexually, we are faced with changes that we don't know how to deal with. At first we are shocked by them, then we don't talk about them and then we are shamed into accepting them as normal, when – and I say this ALL the time – what's common doesn't necessarily equal normal.

Coping with All the Changes

"Give birth." So simple – but for some of us, birth isn't that straightforward. Even a beautiful birth feels a little hard done by when described by those two short words. In fact, most of the pregnancy, birth and postnatal journey feels so much more life-changing than language allows.

I thought I'd prepared for it. But once I'd entered motherhood, I struggled to come to terms with my new identity there. I struggled to come to terms with my new identity in motherhood ("Who am I now?"), with the lack of knowledge I had as a mother ("What the fuck am I doing?") and how a baby works ("What the hell do I do with it?"), and with the huge insecurity I now found I had.

I felt insecure about my body and its appearance, how it now worked and what I should do to rehabilitate; I also didn't know whether I could trust my pelvic floor, or what the impact of my scarring would be, and this "unknowing" meant that I didn't feel able to trust the body that I'd had for nearly 30 years. My mind joined in and threw me a curveball of postnatal depression, rage and mild PTSD from the birth. All of this added up to have a pretty negative impact on my marriage and happiness . . . don't worry, there is a happy ending, but I want to tell you how it all went down first, so that you know that I know how it feels.

My Story

I was lucky to become pregnant quickly, coming off the pill to try (very speculatively) for a baby and getting pregnant very soon afterwards. In fact, I didn't have a period before I saw the little blue lines. Which meant I didn't realise I was pregnant until about eight weeks in. Surprise!

Given how much our bodies and hormones can be thrown out of whack by hormonal medications (if you want an amazing read on this, go to *Period Power* by Maisie Hill), I look back on this now as a minor miracle.

As the owner of a newly minted bump-in-waiting, I tried to keep fit and healthy. Pre-pregnancy, I'd loved moving, and I assumed that wasn't going to stop because I was pregnant. I found I was more tired than before and sometimes couldn't face exercise, when I would have lapped it up before. I felt guilty about this – the first of many things I'd feel guilty about in motherhood. My movement motivation naturally waned further in the third trimester. But in general my approach to exercise was like my approach to pregnancy overall – I carried on regardless, vaguely ignoring the growing bump, and certainly didn't engage with the fact that at some point, I was going to have to give birth.

With my changing body and feelings (hello, hormones) I started to feel I was losing sight of myself and my identity, which I hated. The way that I felt constantly nauseated, the way that being pregnant affected my ability to do things annoyed me. I was irritated by the sheer tiredness, and angry at the way that something that is supposedly so natural could make me feel so hideous. I certainly couldn't appreciate it as the miracle of life. I definitely didn't have a pregnancy glow.

One of the wonderful things about being in a long-term relationship is how comfortable you are with each other. You evolve from strangers to best friends; you know everything about each other and you're okay with that. You're no longer worried about being seen naked, you pee in front of them and you might even (god forbid) fart. But alongside that sense of ease, you might also get a little lazy. Perhaps you make less effort, or become complacent in your intimacy. For me and Bryn, my husband, we didn't cultivate romance enough.

While I had wavered on the "having a baby" question before getting pregnant, Bryn was keener to start a family. I would go from hugely enthusiastic and excited about turning the page to the next chapter, to worrying about whether it was the right time, whether we could cope and how my body would meet the challenge. Bryn is brilliant at reading me and has great emotional intelligence and sensitivity, so he didn't want to pressure me either way, letting me take my time. But my uncertainty and the space he left for me meant that our passion levels waned in the lead-up to getting pregnant. We were busy, I was unsure and, let's face it, some "getting pregnant" sex can often be a little less fun.

And, given that I hated being pregnant – I kept jealously wondering who these people who loved it were – I wasn't overly keen on having sex while I was. Being ambivalent about *getting* pregnant led to a level of uncertainty when I *was* pregnant. This uncertainty impacted my self-confidence and body image, which

I'd only recently found peace with. Entering a new and unknown phase in my life caused me to forget all the lessons I'd learned and fall back to the insecurities I'd grown up with. For me, how I feel about my body is an integral part of being comfortable in myself and enjoying sex, so it was a tricky time to navigate. I don't know any woman who hasn't considered this on some level; it's a tough combination.

When I finally made it through the nine (let's face it, nearer ten) months of pregnancy, my labour was long. I started feeling tightening on Tuesday, but my daughter finally arrived on Friday night. Although the contractions didn't really kick off until the Wednesday, the beginning stages are wearing and didn't allow me to sleep very well! I was exhausted by Friday. The labour was made longer, I think, by my subconscious denial of what my body was going through, and my mental reaction to it. I was scared, super scared. I knew I had to go through the birth, of course (how else was the baby going to come out?), but my body was fighting it. I was stressed, anxious and my muscles were tight. The cortisol was blocking the oxytocin that's needed to help the labour progress. I was so tightly wound that the changes and transitions of birth, which require our powerful uterine and cervical muscles to flex and flow to do their thing, took far longer than they would otherwise have done. Those of you who took hypnobirthing classes, which I didn't the first time round, will remember this.

I started off in the midwife-led suite of the labour ward, with naive plans for a nice pool to birth in and a double bed waiting for us to snuggle up in as a family of three after she was born, but it wasn't meant to be.

Having had gas and air and not feeling an impact at all, I soon requested pethidine.[2] One of the side effects of using pethidine for pain relief can be drowsiness, which meant that I then couldn't get into the birthing pool anyway – falling asleep in water isn't a great idea – so bang went that option. I struggled through for another hour, uncertain what I wanted to do; I didn't have a fixed birth plan as I'd wanted to stay open and not be disappointed if things didn't go as planned. In hindsight, perhaps I would have been better suited to writing out a more concrete birth plan.

I eventually requested an epidural, for which I needed to move to the obstetrician-led part of the ward. This move coincided with a change in midwife shift, so it took longer than expected. When I was finally checked in through the other side of the double doors, the anaesthetists changed shift too, so it was even longer before anyone came to see me about the epidural.

Then our baby's heart rate kept dropping – and you need a steady trace (heartbeat) in order to be given an epidural, so I still didn't get one. The heart rate kept dropping and reappearing, which was due (I later found out) to the umbilical cord being around her neck and essentially strangling her every time she started to descend. Although it's normal for the baby's heart rate to drop during contractions and then get stronger again afterwards, my baby's was taking longer than it should to return to normal. I wrote that quite matter-of-factly, but as I read it back, it does sound quite stark and I feel emotional about it even some years on.

By the time we were at the point of administering the epidural four hours later, I was almost fully dilated anyway. It wouldn't have been worth giving it, as it might have slowed things down at the final hurdle. But as I started to push, my baby wouldn't descend to be born. The cord was too short, or perhaps I wasn't pushing effectively. But something wasn't right, and she wasn't coming out.

So I climbed up to lie on the bed in stirrups. I wanted to be mobile, but my midwife preferred me to be on my back and raised up so the medical team could see properly. The obstetrician tried a ventouse[3] delivery (which didn't work) and then an episiotomy and forceps[4] (which did) to get my daughter out. The episiotomy was stitched up after delivery, and created a scar. The forceps delivery also caused internal grazing to my vaginal wall. Because the cord was too short, the obstetrician needed to untangle it from her neck once the head had crowned, but as she did so, it snapped. I'm told that blood went everywhere! But due to the blood loss, my baby had to be resuscitated. I held her for ten seconds before she was whisked away to the neonatal intensive care unit (NICU) for a blood transfusion; she stayed there for four days.

This introduction to motherhood was tough, though I didn't overthink it at the time – we do what we need to to get through. And there are plenty of other people in worse situations, right? The episiotomy scar and forceps graze would both be relevant to my journey back to postnatal sexual health, but at the time all I wanted was to drink the cup of tea I was offered.

Physical Changes

I don't know if you noticed, but when you grow a baby and push it out, your body changes. Not just a little, but a lot. It's a big deal, growing an actual human being inside your own body. Pretty incredible when you think about it.

So let's do that. Stop and think about it properly. Firstly, to make way for this new human, your organs literally have to get out of the way. Your ribs move up and out, your stomach and lungs are squashed up, your bladder and digestive system are pushed down, your pelvic floor carries a few extra kilos of weight on it and your skin (yes, that's an organ too) stretches to accommodate a bowling-ball-sized baby. This is awe-inspiring stuff.

And because these are quite intense shifts, it does mean that we have some way to go to resume normal business afterwards. Makes sense, right? But so often we don't give ourselves the time or space to do that. We feel like we need to pick up exactly where we left off pre-pregnancy, as if the pregnancy and birth didn't happen at all.

This isn't your fault – due to the constant narrative of judgement of women's bodies that we have playing in our heads, we feel the need to act as if nothing has happened. So if you take one thing away from this book, I want you to remember that slow and steady wins the race. This isn't about bouncing back or snapping back into shape. This isn't, in fact, about going back at all. It's about slowly and surely moving forward into your new body and new identity, and acknowledging all the wonderful things you've done.

Your body and your mind are different now. You might be softer in the body, and certainly a little woolly in the mind sometimes (baby brain is real!), and those things are fine. You can embrace this, or you can work to incorporate your new identity into the old and create something completely new. You might come back to running marathons or cross-training four days a week again, and you'll almost certainly be back at work in whatever successful capacity you were before, but you'll do them in a new way. That new way isn't any less, it's just different, and actually sometimes better.

Pelvic Floor Weakness and Pelvic Floor Over-Tightness

Let's start with a very common issue. The weak pelvic floor. I've lost count of the number of times I've heard or seen a mother laugh off incontinence, however slight, after having a baby. They pick up pads with their weekly shopping and think nothing more of it. They ask in running forums which leggings hide accidental wees the best.

These mums don't run or exercise like they used to, or if they do, they have to put up with wetting themselves; they can't safely pick up the pace to catch a bus, and they don't play in the park like they want to with their kids. The pelvic floor muscles have a lot to contend with and some substantial weight to carry while you're pregnant. If you're a mum of twins or multiples, I salute you!

Your set of pelvic floor muscles hold in the organs in your torso. If the pelvic floor wasn't there, your bladder, uterus and bowel would be swinging about in a bag between your legs. The baby grows in your uterus, so when it grows, both the weight and size of the baby ensure the pelvic floor is being pushed down. The pelvic floor muscles form a sort of "figure of eight" shape around three openings – the anus, the vagina and the urethra – so that you can let stuff, mainly waste fluids/matter and penises, in and out. So if you give birth vaginally, the pelvic floor must stretch and move in a different direction to make way for the baby to emerge. All of this is something that it doesn't do very regularly, and if it's a first baby, it might never have done it before (which is why it can take a little longer for first births to progress).

So what does that weight and that massive workout do for your pelvic floor? Well, understandably, it stretches and tires it. Check out our clingfilm video on www.andbreathewellbeing. com/get-your-mojo-back for a great illustration (honestly, it's better than it sounds). This all means that there's a lot of work you might need to do to regain elasticity and strength. That's totally normal, and takes time, but we don't often give ourselves that time or read our bodies to really figure out what they need.

So how to solve this? I know it's boring, but let's talk Kegels. When the midwife quickly asks you if you're doing your pelvic floor exercises, it's important to do more than just nod and think, "well, duh!" Over 50 per cent of us[5] are thought to be doing our pelvic floor exercises incorrectly, which is a staggering figure. This isn't that surprising when you think that most of us aren't ever really taught the proper technique at all, and that even if we have been instructed, it was probably via written instructions or remotely, rather than in conjunction with a physiotherapist. Doing your pelvic floor exercises incorrectly can mean a range of things: it could mean a lack of strength, poor technique, or even (at the extreme) actively bearing down rather than lifting.

What happens if that's you? Well, again there's a range: you might be doing them fine, but just not *as effectively* as you could be. Which means that when you really stress the pelvic floor (perhaps a longer run with more liquids than usual, or sneezing while hopping onto an escalator with hands full of groceries), it might not cope. Perhaps later in life, when muscle tone starts to diminish and elasticity disappears, you might be in trouble.

On the other hand, you might be doing them completely *ineffectively*. Which means that you won't be building up strength or flexibility. Flexibility, as I've mentioned before, is just as important as strength, because if our pelvic floor muscles are too tight, they also can't function properly. We must remember to release as well as lift, and this can be just as difficult to remember as doing the Kegels in the first place!

What's only just coming to light now is that no-one's releasing [the pelvic floor]. People don't realise that pain and the pelvic floor can be connected, and that what's important is to be strong *and* flexible. Your hamstrings and your pelvic floor are both muscles, and you'd always stretch after a workout – how can you wee or poo or have sex if you can't stretch out the muscles as well as tense them?
Amanda Savage, Women's Health Physiotherapist

The good news is that this can all be improved in time – the key is allowing yourself that time and self-love to get there. Think of rehab as a pyramid. It took our bodies nearly ten months to go from the start to the end of pregnancy (to the peak of the pyramid), so it's only sensible that it can take the same amount of time to work to full strength again afterwards.

As we're talking about training a part of the body we can't see, it's not really surprising that our Kegels might be sub-optimal.

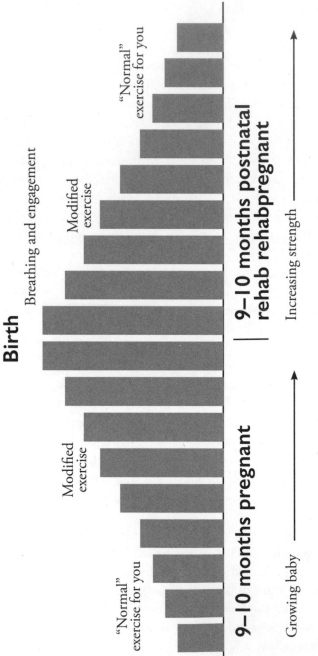

Birth

Breathing and engagement

Modified exercise

"Normal" exercise for you

Modified exercise

"Normal" exercise for you

9–10 months pregnant

9–10 months postnatal rehab rehab pregnant

Growing baby

Increasing strength

Pelvic floor exercises – practice makes perfect!

We often teach ourselves to do them by reading instructions, and even if we're taught to do them in person, it's briskly, and with the details rushed over. If we're reading instructions, there's the added complication of trying to translate written steps into physical movements – which isn't always easy.

So, here's how to do a proper pelvic floor lift:

Top Tips for Pelvic Floor Lifts

- It's not a squeeze, it's a lift. We're imagining slowly pulling a tissue up out of a box, or the aquatic movement of a squid moving through the water: a gentle but strong, flowing and complete movement, not a nipping squeeze.
- During your exercises, when you're lifting, you're lifting to 80 per cent of the maximum.
- After your lift, make sure you RELEASE fully. The pelvic floor is a set of muscles. Muscles need to be equally flexible and strong to work effectively – if you only ever curled your bicep without straightening the arm to stretch the muscle, you'd have great guns, but be unable to move your arm properly. The same goes for your pelvic floor. We need strength *and* flexibility to be able to stop peeing our pants effectively. Who knew?

1. If you're doing these for the first time, it's a good idea to go somewhere quiet and perhaps lie down, so that you can focus. Closing your eyes and sending your thoughts to your pelvic floor (don't laugh) can also be helpful to get you engaging the right muscles.
2. Concentrate on the back part of your pelvic floor (which feels like stopping a fart from coming out). Lift for a slow

count of one, release for a slow count of one, repeat ten
times and hold for a count of five to ten on the last one.

3. Do the same with the front part of your pelvic floor
(which feels like stopping a wee from coming out) and lift
this up for a slow count of one, releasing fully afterwards.
Repeat ten times. Hold the last one for a count of five to
ten (depending on how strong your pelvic floor is and how
newly postnatal you are).

4. Repeat again with the whole pelvic floor area, front and
back. It may help to start at the back (usually the strongest
part) and glide the lift forward to include the front. Lift for
a slow count of one, release for a slow count of one, repeat
ten times and hold for a count of five to ten on the last one.

5. Do this three times per day. If you're busy, you can set a
diary reminder or download an app which helps you to
remember (that's not you, right?!). Don't worry if you forget
them; the beauty of aiming for three times per day is that
you'll hopefully do at least one set. And if you're further
along in motherhood, don't be disheartened – it's never too
late to improve your pelvic floor.

You can gradually build up your lifts in number and length of
hold, and you should be able to see a difference in continence
levels, comfort and strength. Your pelvic floor is an integral part
of your core, so you need it working well to exercise properly
and get functionally strong too. Don't worry if you over-test
it sometimes and you get a little bit of leakage – we need to
stress our body to a certain extent in order to progress. In other
words, if you're not feeling your way to your limits, you won't
know how and where you need to improve or develop your
muscle strength.

Once you've explored the front and back parts of your
pelvic floor, you can see whether you're able to identify the
left and right sides. With concentration and practice, it's
possible to isolate the muscles on each side and lift them by
themselves. You can add this to the cycle of pelvic floor lifts;

for example front, back, left, right, all together. This can be helpful if you have scarring on one side and it's less flexible or more or less sensitive.

Once you've built up your confidence, you can try more nuanced exercises like The Elevator, pelvic floor lifts with different feet positions and mastering The Knack. Visit www.andbreathewellbeing.com/get-your-mojo-back to learn more and for expert guidance.

If you can get a referral or afford it, the best thing is always to check your pelvic floor strength and technique with a women's health physiotherapist , who can do an internal assessment.. As well as helping you to identify whether you're doing them correctly and if you need to focus on building strength or flexibility, they can also identify any referred muscle issues in different parts of your body.

The Word on the Street

Rosalie Genay, singer/songwriter, mum of two

"We generally only get given advice about things like strengthening our pelvic floor, doing our Kegels, etc., but there's not a lot of emphasis on the release part. I was listening to a piece on *Woman's Hour* [on BBC Radio 4] about female athletes with leak problems due to hypertonic pelvic floor which reminded me of this. Like me, a lot of women, either through high-intensity training, sexual trauma or birth trauma have hypertonic pelvic floors, which can result in very similar symptoms to a weak one . . . but until a pelvic floor examination with a women's health physio, I had no idea this was even a thing!"

Core Strength/Weakness and Diastasis Recti

The other obvious set of muscles that really do a great job in pregnancy and postnatally are the abdominal muscles. We're talking about the six-pack and more. Have you ever wondered how a washboard forms? Well it's your lucky day! Your tummy muscles are incredible things.

When we refer colloquially to the "abs", we're normally talking about the rectus abdominis (RA). These are the muscles that run vertically along your stomach, the ones that create that washboard – the showboat muscles. But they're not the only thing at play in a healthily functioning body, and in fact, I'd argue, not the most important ones for women in the postnatal period. That award goes to your other major set of ab muscles, which are called the transverse abdominis (TVA). The TVA runs around your torso like a corset and is a layer below the RA, deeper inside the body. So while the RA is putting on the show, it's the TVA that's doing most of the hard work.

Both the RA and TVA stretch to accommodate the baby (how would it fit otherwise?), and the connective tissue between the two upright sets of RA, called the linea alba, also stretches, which means the rectus abdominis comes apart to a greater or lesser degree. This is normal and is called diastasis rectus abdominis, or DRA, commonly referred to as "ab separation".

What does all this mean? Simple: if your core is feeling loose or weak after you've had a baby, that's only to be expected! Your ab muscles *will* be floppy – they are, after all, much longer than they were before. Again, it takes time to rehabilitate, for the ab muscles to get shorter and stronger and be able to hold tension, and for the ab separation to come together again. At least ten months is a perfectly acceptable timeline for rehabilitation, though if you recover more quickly, that's great, or if it takes more time (and you're seeing progress), that's fine too. But if you haven't rehabilitated sufficiently, a weak ab section can impact the strength of your pelvic floor muscles (they're all linked, don't you know), give you a pouch-y tummy, cause backache and

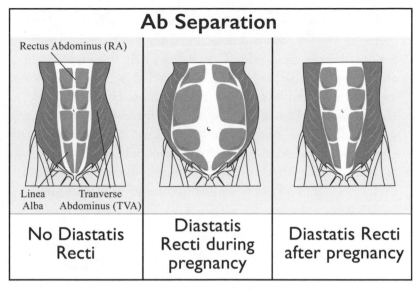

Ab Separation

Rectus Abdominus (RA)

Linea Alba   Tranverse Abdominus (TVA)

| No Diastatis Recti | Diastatis Recti during pregnancy | Diastatis Recti after pregnancy |

From left to right: Rectus abdominis before, during and after pregnancy, showing how ab separation can develop in pregnancy and start to heal as the bump shrinks after birth.

more, especially when coupled with carrying a baby around all-freaking-day.

It's particularly important to focus on healing your diastasis by drawing the RA back together, but that doesn't mean it needs to close completely; many of us will have had a small gap even before pregnancy. Instead, the aim is to lessen the gap as much as you can, but also to build tension underneath. For example, you could have a shallow two-finger gap but with lots of tension behind it, and that would functionally be perfectly fine – we're all different. To close the gap and build tension, we work on strengthening the TVA, which uses its corset shape to draw the core inward and the RA together.

It might sound daunting, but don't worry: a good trainer with experience of pregnancy training and postnatal recovery will be able to set you on the right path with exercises and breathing patterns to get your core engagement going and build up strength. If you're able to have a physiotherapist consultation with an internal examination to assess where you are, all the better. In the UK this can be accessed on the National Health Service (NHS) via a referral from your GP (be prepared to advocate for yourself) or paid for privately (just search for your local women's health physio). I realise this can be a big expense, but it can be worth the outlay to avoid problems worsening down the line and chronic (long-term) issues and pain.

To get you started, there are some great books in the resources at the end of the book, as well as some videos on how to engage the core at www.andbreathewellbeing.com/get-your-mojo-back.

Weight Gain and Stretch Marks

It's completely normal to gain weight while you're pregnant. I gained 10kg (over a stone and a half) on a 153cm (5'1") frame both times. Some of that is baby (which obviously keeps adding more as it grows), some is placenta (hello, it's a whole new organ), some is the fluid inside the uterus and some will be additional fat that you're carrying. All of this adds up, and some of us carry it better than others. Some of us are naturally more inclined to hold on to fat, and we usually gather fat stores of between 2.5 and 4kg during pregnancy. Lots of this is used up during breastfeeding, but unfortunately prolactin (the hormone we produce for breastfeeding) increases appetite as well as helping us to produce milk!

While we might not have to eat for two (thanks, helpful 1950s myth), we often crave more food and the wrong types of food. If you struggled with morning sickness (let's face it, it's never just the morning, is it?), you'll probably have gravitated even more regularly toward junk foods, chocolate, crisps . . . in short, anything that lacks nutritional value but tastes good. I have been there.

Our skin can stretch – it's pretty cool like that – but when it does, it has to incorporate little fissures into its top layers to allow a bit more give and stop itself breaking. These clever little fissures are what we know as stretch marks. But I like to call them tiger stripes. Because I'm a badass, and so are you.

So we're bigger than we were and our smooth skin has changed. To an extent, skin is elastic and can shrink back (with time, of course – I think you know the score by now.) But you might still be left with some more pliable skin and juicier flesh, and that's okay. I know it's hard when the baby is screaming and you're sleep deprived to the max, but remember the amazing feat you've just accomplished. Yes, there are creams, oils and balms you can slather on yourself, and there are supplements, like collagen, that you can take; these are expensive, and, though they might have some effect, they're not miracle workers. It's better to invest time and thought into good nutrition and a balanced diet, which will help balance hormones and give you more restful sleep (when you can get it) and more energy, as well as helping your body build and protect itself. But I only want you to do this with love in your heart for your body. What will really help is working with your body, not against it. Embrace those changes and pour love into your body, and that's when you'll start to see the difference.

Weight gain, tiger stripes, wrinkles, wobbly bits, pliable skin . . . we're made to feel bad about all of them, but for me the power is found in rethinking our beauty ideals and taking ownership of what is ours in the first place. One great voice of many in this arena is Alex Light, whose book *You Are Not a Before Picture* is a must-read. Who says all those things are not desirable? Let's turn that dialogue around and embrace them. Look, I know it's not easy. You might not want to, you might find it hard to engage with this conversation and with your body. You might tell me to eff off. That's okay too, as long as you're listening to what I'm saying, and questioning the old dialogue, or even just recognising that you are allowed to question it. Think about this. My friend's daughter ran out of the bathroom after seeing her mum get out of the shower. She came back with a pen to draw stripes on her own body, like stretch marks, because she wanted to "be like mummy". That's pretty cool too, isn't it?

Your Breasts

Well, we can't talk about body changes without touching on the ladies now, can we? The development and appearance of our boobs are part and parcel of our journey into womanhood, and the changes they undergo as we become mothers are even more amazing, and sometimes unexpected. They'll probably be all over the place during pregnancy: sensitive, tender, swollen and bigger than usual. That's nothing compared to their shenanigans postpartum. When milk comes in, they might be rock-hard and painful, and during your breastfeeding journey they could feel full, empty, sore, itchy, blistered and cracked. Our nipples take a hell of a sucking. Our breasts usually remain bigger than normal until we stop breastfeeding; then they revert to their usual size, or for some women perhaps a touch smaller. They might remain perky or be a little flatter.

You might want them touched, but many of us don't, which can be an issue if they had been a primary part of sex for you previously. If you are breastfeeding, it can be confusing too to experience the rush of oxytocin when you "let down", the very same hormone that we usually associate with love and can feel a lot during sex. Practically speaking, those boobs might also want to spray a load of milk around during sex too, which, depending on your inclination, might not be everyone's cup of tea . . .

The good news is that, as with most physical changes we experience, it doesn't have to be permanent. Once you stop breastfeeding, your breasts' sensitivity will revert back to pre-baby levels and you can start to think of them as the reliable sexual protagonists they once were. Even if you are able and choose to continue to breastfeed for a number of years, your body will adapt over time to enable them to play a dual role for you. Clever them.

Hair and Skin

You might have been one of the lucky ones who actually did get a pregnancy glow, but for those of us who heaved over the toilet bowl, it wasn't so apparent. Either way, we're pumping a whole lot more blood around our bodies when we're pregnant, and post-birth that takes a while to dissipate; hormones are out of whack and you're sleep deprived and probably not eating the most healthy choices. All of which means your skin might take a hammering. I had spots a-go-go and still have two dark patches (melasma) on my upper lip that added to my "with-it" new-mum look. It was almost like being a teenager again, except I definitely couldn't stay in bed until noon.

You also keep hold of your hair when pregnant, which can mean it feels fuller and more lustrous, but also means that postnatally you'll find a lot of that dropping out. Don't worry, you're not going bald, but you might have to unblock that shower drain a little more regularly than usual; this, along with your skin, will regulate itself after a few months, but in the interim, it's understandable if you don't feel at your sexiest!

Scarring (Vaginal and C-Section)

I've talked about scarring and how it can affect sensation. But what causes scars in the first place? Scar tissue builds up where broken tissue knits together. The tissue fibres knit in a messy criss-cross pattern, kind of like a tangled ball of string, laying down new material wherever they can in order to heal the wound as quickly and securely as possible, rather than in neat orderly lines following the path of existing tissue. Scars are an amazing function of the body, but often the way that the scar tissue is laid down can mean that it's bulky and doesn't lie flat. It means that the wound is safe and closed, but the bulky or too-tight tissue can also pull surrounding tissues and muscles in new directions, causing aches and pains, tightness, soreness and overhang where they didn't exist before. Over time, with massage, you can add suppleness to the scar tissue fibres so that they are more inclined to give in the direction of the original fibres, but we rarely get told this or are given the information to practise it ourselves.

Get Your Mojo Back 101

Hannah Johnson – sports massage therapist and C-section scar specialist @hannahjohnsontherapies

"The way I like to describe it is that scar tissue is like the body's cement. When you have a wound or a trauma to the body, its main aim is to stick you back together as quickly as possible. So when you've had a caesarean, your body just wants to put itself back together, and it lays down the scar tissue, which like cement is very sticky and hard. It just wants to keep everything closed and protected from infection. You actually have layers and layers of tissue that have been cut to get a caesarean baby out, so that scar tissue is also going all the way through those layers: it's not just what we see on the surface of the tummy, but it's going all the way down to the uterus. People sometimes forget there's a lot going on underneath: I liken it to an iceberg – what we see on the tummy is just the tip, and underneath is much more far-reaching than we can see. I tell people to massage their whole tummy because it's not just the visible scar line that we need to work on – under the surface it could be affecting everything.

Scar tissue doesn't form lines uniformly. It goes wherever it wants, and it will stick to whatever it comes into contact with – it doesn't discriminate, because it just wants to secure the wound. With major abdominal surgery like a C-section, it has the potential to stick to your intestines, your bowel, your reproductive organs . . . and this hard scar tissue can cause problems later on.

Underneath the skin, we've got a connective tissue called fascia which covers our whole body. I liken it to a wetsuit: you're wearing this whole-body suit, but every part of it is like a web and it goes in between organs and muscles everywhere, and it's all linked into one big organ. Imagine that if you're wearing something tight like a wetsuit, you feel it in all different places. If it's tight on your shoulder, you might also feel it down on your hip. Another way to think of it is like those parachutes at toddler groups, with everyone holding on around the edge. If you're on one end and someone's pulling from the other side, you can feel it pulling in your hands as well. So when you have a scar, if you think of it as tissue being pulled or bunched up at one end, you're definitely going to feel it somewhere else in the body. But we don't often make that connection: if you've got a tight jaw or neck, you don't necessarily think that's coming from your scar. But it absolutely has the potential to be coming from that: anything that disrupts our fascia in some way (like scar tissue) is going to be affecting other parts of the body as well.

That's where massage comes in. It can help to prevent the build-up of that scar tissue. If we just leave the body to its own devices, in some people it will be fine. But in the majority of women, they will notice something: some pain, some numbness, a feeling of restriction or pulling, and that is where that scar tissue is tight and pulling on the fascia. With the massage, we're trying to provide movement to those tissues; where that cement just wants to stay stuck and still, we just want to give it a bit more flexibility. I don't believe that we can 'break down' scar tissue, what we're doing is just helping it to function in your body better and have a bit more movement. That might also mean helping the tissues around the scar tissue to be more flexible, which in turn helps the scar tissue itself to be more flexible. With massage you're also helping those tissues to get oxygen and better blood flow, and in turn that's helping to reduce pain, numbness and feelings of restriction.

Desensitisation can be a great place to start massage. Often people can experience both hypersensitivity and numbness, which seems a contradiction but is really common. A lot of women find it hard to touch or to look at their scars to start with. So desensitisation using gentle touch with a make-up brush or cotton ball helps them to get used to the new emotional feelings and physical sensations, and also improves that numbness. Because I think numbness, apart from obviously the physical changes that are occurring, can also be due to the mental connection (or disconnection) with our tummy. The body to make new neural pathways between the brain and tummy after pregnancy, for both caesarean and vaginal births, so massage and desensitisation are part of that. The nerves themselves regrow within the first five to seven days, but your brain takes longer to adapt.

With C-section recovery massage, I probably work more around the scar than I do on it. We can get very fixated on having to release the scar, and this is where all the tension is, but I find, for example, that people's hips can be really tight, and when we loosen the hips off, actually the scar softens. I work right up to the ribs and the diaphragm – the whole core, really, down to the pelvis, is so important.

When it comes to massage, there's always this misconception that it has to be painful to be beneficial. Softer techniques can be so much better, because we want the body to feel safe enough to relax, we want it to let go of things and to work with us; we're actually working on the nervous system, which impacts the whole body, and I'm more of a facilitator to help that happen in a way.

It's really important to make sure you think of your body as a whole. Movement, even getting out for a walk or stretching, is going to benefit your body's healing. We spend a lot of time in the initial postpartum days being hunched over: feeding, sleeping positions, carrying things. And if we're bent over and our scar is healing

> in that way, then it's going to be even tighter. So just remembering to open up our chest and gently lean back, even in the early days, giving that space to the tummy as well, is really important. Movement is a massive part of helping your scar to stay supple."

Desensitising scars and making them more supple is a long process, but slow and steady wins the race, like in many other kinds of rehabilitation. The great thing about this process is that you can do a lot yourself, especially once you've been shown the basics. A good women's health physio and/or postnatal massage specialist will be able to look at and assess your internal and C-section scars with touch, as well as helping you understand the impact they're having on surrounding tissue and where there is tightness or sensitivity, and giving you the exercises and movements and massage techniques to help improve these.

Scar Massage Basics

Hannah Johnson says that her first step is always breathing: "Become aware of *where* you're breathing, put your hand on your scar or just above, and just focus on breathing down into the abdomen as far as you can. Most women breathe a lot in their chests, protecting that tummy, and avoiding the lower part of the belly." We often get into this protective mode of breathing while we're healing, so learning that it's good to breathe more fully is the first step. Then:

1. Start with allowing your body to relearn any sensation by brushing your fingers lightly over your scar once it's healed (usually around six weeks postpartum). You can do this in the shower or lying on your back in bed (before you collapse into exhausted sleep!). In the shower is great so that you can

build the habit, and in bed is great so that your core is fully relaxed when you're doing it. If you're doing it in the shower, take a few deep breaths before you start the massage to make sure the muscles are as relaxed as they can be.

2. You might feel emotional doing this, or even at the thought of doing this, and that's common too. Don't push yourself to address your scar before you're ready. Once you are, a softly-softly approach is best in order to gently probe the sensations and feelings associated with your scarring and birth. It will get better in time as you process and come to terms with anything that's coming up for you.

3. Start to use other objects, such as ribbons, feathers or a small ball, to brush and roll over the tissue. The different objects produce different sensations, which again helps your brain to reconnect with your nervous system and in turn helps the tissues to relax and rehabilitate. You can also massage the abdomen, hips and quads – and the areas around the scar/pelvis too – and you might want to do this more firmly, even from an earlier stage. Just be aware not to pull too much on the scar itself.

4. When you feel able (and always after the wound is fully healed, generally after six weeks) you can start to apply more pressure directly to the scar and to the surrounding tissue. Remember that we're not trying to massage the scar into submission though! This is a slow journey, and it's not supposed to be painful.

5. Use a natural oil to help your fingers glide, so that you are not pulling so much on the skin as you massage. Oils such as coconut oil, or a favourite of mine, cold-pressed organic rose hip oil, which also contains a lot of vitamin E, are great options – it doesn't have to be a specific scar product.

6. What movements should I use? Hannah suggests these:
   - Broad sweeps with the fingers, hand or even inner arm, back and forth above, below and on the scar.
   - Circles with your fingers, moving left to right and back again, above, below and on the scar.

- Zig-zagging up and down over the top of the scar.
- Gently manipulate the tissue above and below the scar to pull the scar up and down, to encourage movement in the scar tissue.
- Roll the scar and the surrounding tissue gently in your fingers.
- Check out our videos on www.andbreathewellbeing.com/get-your-mojo-back for demos.

7. You may also want to wear a silicone band on top of the scar, which can really help with a raised or red scar, particularly if used up to 18 months postnatal.

Remember that these scars can affect parts of the body other than just the scar itself, so you might be wondering where the pain in your hips or glutes is coming from, without realising that your C-section scar is too tight. It makes sense, really, doesn't it? A caesarean is major abdominal surgery, and we are left with layers of healing. The scar is usually more than 10cm (3.9") long,[6] so it should be no surprise that it impacts other surrounding parts of the body. Don't forget that this is all part of the journey; it's nothing you've done wrong and is completely normal – it's just that we seem to not be given scar rehab advice after a caesarean like we might after other operations. You can see improvement very quickly for some symptoms (eg pain or tightness), but others will take longer – and as Hannah says, "Consistency is key!"

Hormones Affect Breastfeeding, Libido and Lubrication!

In case all of that wasn't enough to deal with, our hormones, though they are damned clever little things, can cause us a touch of havoc too. Hormones are the little chemical messengers that race around our bodies telling each bit what to do. They are incredibly helpful, but when there are big changes in our bodies, there are correspondingly big changes in hormone levels, which can mean that things are out of whack for a little while.

The main hormones in the postnatal period are: prolactin, the breastfeeding hormone; oxytocin, the love hormone; relaxin, the flexi hormone; and oestrogen, also known (to me, anyway) as the mother of all hormones.

- **Prolactin:** Increases dramatically after birth, as this is the hormone that stimulates breastfeeding. It can also stimulate hunger, so that you eat enough food to provide milk for your baby (which also makes those cravings hard to ignore), but doesn't necessarily tell you when to stop eating.
- **Oxytocin:** A big player during the birth as well as postpartum, this hormone makes you feel all the feels and bond with your baby. During the birth it helps your uterus contract, and it also helps it to shrink again afterwards. It stimulates the let down of breastfeeding, but is also likely to be present during intimacy. So it can cause milk-spraying boobs at the most inopportune moments.
- **Relaxin:** The hormone that relaxes ligaments in preparation for childbirth; it enables your pelvis to move and allow the baby's head through. It can remain high through postpartum and breastfeeding, which means you can feel wobblier than usual. Affects balance and what exercise you feel able to do. This in turn can have an impact on your confidence and sensuality.
- **Oestrogen:** Drops sharply post birth, and remains low if you are breastfeeding. This is why you won't have a period for a while, and when your period does return (usually as you start to breastfeed less or after stopping breastfeeding), it's a sign that your oestrogen levels are returning to normal. Low levels can also cause vaginal tenderness and dryness (lack of lubrication), which can make sex painful. The medical term for this is vaginal atrophy, but I think that sounds scarier and more accusatory than it needs to, so just pick up some organic lube and go with it for now – lube is your friend! We'll talk more about lube and other gadgets in Chapter 7.

Get Your Mojo Back 101

Dr Brooke Vandermolen – obstetrics and gynaecology registrar @theobgynmum

"There is a tremendous focus on the run up to birth: deep thought and preparation about getting pregnant, gentle hypnobirthing to prepare for labour. But very rarely does anyone talk about the seismic changes that happen postpartum. The delicate hormonal balance that allows a complex process like pregnancy to occur, whereby your body tolerates and nurtures a foreign body inside of your own, means that the levels of key hormones such as progesterone and oestrogen are altered, and this has a wide range of effects. After pregnancy is over, these levels change to allow breastfeeding to occur, and later they fully correct themselves so that fertility can return when the menstrual cycle resumes again. These hormonal changes cause many effects which can be difficult to tolerate: mood changes, insomnia, irregular bleeding, dry skin, sleep disturbance, the list goes on. Forewarned is forearmed, so if women were better prepared, it might be easier to adjust to the process.

It's normal for the vagina to feel drier than usual after childbirth. This is linked to the lower levels of oestrogen in your body compared to when you were pregnant. Levels of oestrogen are lower in breastfeeding mothers than in those who aren't breastfeeding, and the dryness can be more marked. Once you stop breastfeeding and your periods have returned, the levels of oestrogen revert to pre-pregnancy levels and normal vaginal moisturisation is usually restored. Vaginal dryness can be uncomfortable and can lead to pain during intercourse. It is, however, easy to treat and manage, so don't hesitate to seek advice.

There's a physical reason for the dip in sex drive that happens postpartum. When a woman is pregnant, her reproductive hormones are elevated, and after giving birth they crash. This results in a dip in oestrogen and testosterone, which can cause low sex drive and vaginal dryness, making sex feel painful. It is like an evolutionary mechanism to ensure that she takes the time to properly heal and focus on caring for the baby instead of on trying to have another one. High oxytocin levels during the bonding and breastfeeding process can replace some of the urge to connect intimately through sex.

Even later in motherhood, the reality is that a mother's body has drastically changed, and can feel unrecognisable to her. This is then paired with stress and anxiety about keeping her baby alive and doing everything 'right'! At the same time, and even long after the postnatal phase, she is exhausted, overwhelmed and seriously sleep deprived. This can contribute to pushing sex and intimacy lower down the list of priorities, even as the hormonal changes correct themselves."

A Note on the Perimenopause

If low oestrogen and hormone imbalance symptoms last past the postnatal and early parenthood phase, or you feel that the symptoms are a lot worse than you should be experiencing, you may be shifting into the perimenopause or starting to see signs of pre-perimenopause. The pre-perimenopause is what I call the changes and fluctuations that many of us start to experience in our hormone levels past the age of 35. It's a bit of a tongue-twister, and it's a bit like the trailer before the main movie of the perimenopause – in that it lets you know what joys are in store! Like a lot of things in life, the perimenopause is not a clearcut period, but a phase which builds up gradually. When the postnatal period and the hormone transition around perimenopause occur at the same time, it can mean that the impact of those hormone shifts is even greater.

Until 2020, the birth rate for women over 40 was the only growing birth rate category in the UK,[9] so if this is you, you're not alone. It's worth talking to your GP, keeping track of your moods and physical changes to track your hormone levels and/ or paying for hormone testing privately. By observing and monitoring our bodies, we can go into the perimenopause and menopausal (post-period) phase forewarned and forearmed, ready to embrace the next new stage of our amazing bodies.

Mental Ch-Ch-Ch-Changes

These physical changes can affect us mentally too. It is, after all, a pretty tough time to be going through. Even if you aren't diagnosed with anything specific, feeling low, anxious, ragey and, well, just a bit off are all completely normal. But what else might we be dealing with?

Postnatal Depression and Other Mood Disorders

Postnatal depression (or postpartum depression) has been around forever, but previous generations weren't quite as open about it as we are now. Even now, we might share more with close friends and family, but in public we tend to sweep things under the carpet a little and pretend we're getting on fine. But over one in ten women experience postnatal depression or postnatal anxiety[7] (often two ends of the same symptom spectrum) and over half of women experience the baby blues[8] (temporary low mood which can occur a few days after birth). The baby blues will go away on its own, but if you are still experiencing symptoms after two weeks, you should seek help and advice from your GP, as some parents may need talking therapy or medication to support their recovery from postnatal depression and/or anxiety. At the far end of the scale is postpartum psychosis, affecting 1 in 1,000 women[10]: symptoms can include hallucinations and delusions, and it can be incredibly scary for all involved. Treatment is usually as an in-patient at a specialist mother and baby mental health ward. While it can be extremely worrying at the time, mothers who experience this usually go on to make a full recovery.

There is no firm cause of postnatal depression and other mood disorders. Factors include previous mental health history, biological triggers (research is ongoing into hormonal triggers, eg stopping breastfeeding), change in lifestyle (ahem, a new baby perhaps), stress on your relationship (see again, new baby), stressful life events (er . . . new baby?) and comparative images of motherhood (I'm looking at you, Instagram). But like any time of great change, it's only natural that childbirth might impact us in some way – especially if we have previous experience of mental health issues, as I did. These mental health conditions, whether they're mild or more serious, can have an impact on our everyday lives, how we feel about ourselves and our relationships, and therefore on sex and intimacy.

You can visit the mental health charity Mind (www.mind.org.uk) for a comprehensive overview of perinatal mental health issues. There is also a great list of Chapter 2 resources at the end of the book for further reading and help. If you think you might need more support with your mental health, do see your GP or seek advice from another medical professional such as your midwife or health visitor, who should be able to refer you on for counselling if needed.

Old vs New: Identity and Body Image

We can struggle with the change between our old, comfortable and *known* identity and the new identity that we find ourselves with. Babies mean a change of routine, moving into unfamiliar territory, not knowing what we're doing and navigating a new landscape in our relationships with lovers as well as with friends and family. That's a lot to deal with, and not all of us take to it well.

The transition to motherhood encompasses our physical self too. We become used to how we look in the mirror, how our clothes fit and how we move. Often, how we view ourselves is something we've been working on for a lifetime! So when pregnancy, and then childbirth, and then the existence of a baby in your life wreaks havoc on that, it's okay if you find it difficult to find your balance again. It probably won't happen immediately, at least.

We can find ourselves wondering how we'll cope with our new bodies, fixating on how to get back to our old one and, yes, not feeling too great about any changes. But it's worth bearing in mind the pressures that we've grown up under and become accustomed to – starting with the way that the media portrays and judges women's bodies, and the trickle-down effect that has on our own self-judgement and shame.

When we're in an unfamiliar body, it's entirely expected that we might feel uncomfortable, but that doesn't have to last. Rather than listening to cultural pressures to look entirely like we haven't had a baby, you could instead lean into the wonder of your body, whatever it looks like. It has, after all, carried you, carried and birthed a baby (or babies), moved, danced, lived, travelled, loved and more. It's not easy to make peace with that against the background of (ugh) "bouncing back", but it is possible. And if you want some company and encouragement, there are more and more wonderful examples of women who are doing it their way and embracing themselves and whatever shape, size and colour they are. Natalie Lee (@stylemesunday), Danae Mercer (@danaemercer) and Alex Light (@alexlight_ldn) are all brilliant Instagram accounts to follow.

Birth Fear and Birth Trauma

If we've experienced a traumatic birth, the impact of this on our long-term mental health can also be unexpected. Remember that trauma doesn't have to meet a minimum goriness threshold – it's simply a question of how you experience it. I hear so many women refer to their births with the words, "oh but it wasn't that bad, so many others have it worse" or "but it's all alright now!" I understand why you would, I've said them myself. But it's also okay not to minimise your experience in the face of what others have been through: all our experiences are valid.

This book is not a deep dive into birth trauma – for that I can recommend Emma Svanberg's *Why Birth Trauma Matters* and the other resources for this chapter at the end of the book – but it's important to mention its impact on your broader postnatal mental health. If we have experienced trauma, the need to protect ourselves can affect our conscious or subconscious physical reactions to being touched, intimacy, penetration and more. You may not be ready for penetrative sex for a while. You may not be ready for *any* level of intimacy for a while.

You might even be experiencing post-traumatic stress disorder (PTSD). Usually associated with war veterans, this can be the body's reaction to any traumatic experience, which, depending on your birth and mental health situation, could be mild to severe. However, it's much more common to experience birth trauma without PTSD, so don't be alarmed!

These birth reactions can feel overwhelming and impossible to solve, but for the majority of women they can be resolved, given enough time, patience and self-compassion. Talking to your partner or a trusted friend or family member, or someone else in your support network, to let them know how you're feeling and reacting is key, to ease any pressure you might be feeling to jump straight back under the covers. It's best to be honest so that whoever is offering you a friendly ear and support can be as helpful as possible. You can also find some amazing virtual support groups online such as "The Village – Parenting Community" on Facebook. It's also important to establish whether you need further talking therapy either via your GP or privately.

A great place to start for more information is the Birth Trauma Association, www.birthtrauma.org.uk. If you think you might need more support with birth trauma, do visit your GP or seek advice from another medical professional such as your midwife or health visitor.

Hormones and the Emotional Rollercoaster

We talked about these clever little devils just a few pages ago, but they bear mentioning again here, because although we often refer to the body and mind as two separate entities, they are obviously linked and both form part of what makes us, us. Our hormones race around as physical chemicals in our bodies, but their impact is felt both physically and mentally. Whatever your low mood – from the baby blues to anything more serious, and from simple fatigue to confusion and overwhelm – it's normal to feel a little lost and discombobulated after you've had a baby, and let's face it, even into parenthood in the longer term. This means that, for some of us, sex just doesn't feature as much as it once did. We don't find ourselves in that mental space or have time for our relationships or ourselves – and that time is a key building block of intimacy.

How Does This All Link to Our Libido?

All of these factors can contribute to low libido or sexual reluctance or even fear of intimacy. Our bodies can mount campaigns against us, knowing us better than we know ourselves. We might proclaim ourselves ready for sex, but the unconscious tightening of our pelvic floor muscles (vaginismus) might beg to differ. Sometimes the fine balance that we've established over many years of growing into our adult identities is particularly hard to get back, and we just don't feel in the right headspace for sex, let alone at one with and sexy in our bodies. We're tired, wired and stressed (hello cortisol), which is not conducive to feeling sexy.

Any and all of the issues I've been describing in this chapter have symptoms that can impact our sex drive: apathy or lethargy (not great for any activity, let alone sexy time); over or undereating (the associated feelings it might bring up, feeling too full to want to get jiggy); anger (not ideal for romance); uncontrolled black mood (ditto); in fact any mental health experience is likely to push all thoughts of sex onto the back burner! It's completely understandable that sex just isn't the same experience that we would expect pre-pregnancy. And that's what I'm here to help you navigate.

The Word on the Street

Lavinia Winch, 70, women's health champion and lubrication expert, mum of three and grandmother of six

"I fell in love with my first boyfriend at 16, and having received no sex education from my parents and only able to pick up vague references from friends, I realise now that I was hopelessly unprepared for the physical side of our relationship. We muddled along, and after at least a year of tenderness and fumbling, I visited the Brook Advisory Centre with my boyfriend. Brook took a very progressive approach to young people's sexual health, and it was agreed I should take the contraceptive pill. What no one told me at the time, and I have only recently become aware of this myself, is that the pill can cause vaginal dryness due to the change in hormone levels.

In 1969 there was no Google to conveniently search for information on soreness, irritation and painful sex, all of which were distressing. The choice was to go to your doctor (usually a male GP) and be brave enough to explain extremely intimate symptoms and ask for help, or go to an STD clinic to find out if symptoms were due to thrush or another STD. Frequent visits to the doctor or clinic would result in my being told I had thrush and being given some anti-fungal cream to cure the yeast infection. Not surprisingly, my sex life was not very fulfilling and certainly far removed from the wild, passionate and adventurous experiences everyone else seemed to be having! Looking back on these times, I feel sad that my early sexual experiences were so hindered by ignorance and a lack of knowledge or public awareness of the problems associated with the pill.

In 1976 I came off the pill and had a copper coil inserted. With a wonderfully supportive partner my sex life gradually improved, and, being young and in love, we married in 1978. We were blissfully happy and at last I felt able to express myself sexually, as I was free of the symptoms that had made it so difficult. After about 18 months we decided to start a family and the coil was removed. Our daughter was born in 1980, and the episiotomy and many stitches that I had were considered to be fairly normal for many women. The joy our new daughter brought us outweighed any discomfort as we settled down to be new parents.

After six weeks it was clear that I was in no fit state to be making love again. The episiotomy had caused severe scarring, and any attempts were abandoned as it was too painful. The need for some additional lubrication to lessen the discomfort of penetration led us to KY jelly – it had become the label of preference as a sexual lubricant. In the 1980s there was no other brand available, and as far as I know, anyone who needed lubrication would use Vaseline, Baby Oil or KY. At this time there was little information available about ingredients in personal care and cosmetic products, and I was certainly not aware of the side effects of using these products on the sensitive mucous membranes of the vagina.

It never occurred to me that these symptoms could be caused by the use of a lubricant, and no doctor ever suggested that this could be part of the problem. In fact, even an eminent Harley Street dermatologist with a special interest in vulval dermatology was unable to give a satisfactory diagnosis for my condition. I had a biopsy, which revealed nothing, and on further visits to specialists I was advised not to use soap for washing, to shower instead of having baths, to stop wearing tights in the summer, to use only non-bio washing powder and to only wear knickers with cotton gussets. Finally, one dermatologist told me not to wear any black underwear because the dye could cause irritation! Eventually, I was told I had vulval eczema and was prescribed stronger and stronger steroid ointments and creams. I was concerned about the use of steroids because they can thin the skin, and this didn't seem to be a great idea for the most intimate area of my body.

When I used the creams and refrained from having sex, the symptoms would very gradually disappear until we were able to have sex again, with added KY, and then the problems would start all over again! I just didn't have the knowledge to be able to understand what was happening.

Like many women, I also suffered from fairly frequent urinary tract infections. I now know that these infections, like thrush, are more likely to occur when the pH balance of the vagina is disrupted. The frequent use of a glycerine-based lubricant can affect the delicately balanced pH of a healthy vagina, so this was another problem I had to deal with. Further research has helped me to understand that vaginal dryness is often associated with elevated vaginal pH, and elevated vaginal pH increases the likelihood of infections. So using a correctly pH-balanced lubricant brings the vaginal pH back to its protective acidic levels. Using a lubricant that contains small amounts of glycerine can feed thrush, and using a lubricant primarily based on glycerine or glycols will irritate the sensitive vaginal tissues; normal lovemaking can cause damage to these tissues, allowing infections to take hold. So it's a vaginal double whammy if I use a glycerine-based lubricant with a pH above 5.5!

As I approached the menopause in my early fifties, the dryness problems became worse, and I considered hormone replacement therapy (HRT) as a way of helping these symptoms. With no history of breast cancer in my family, I decided that my quality of life was being severely affected and that I was prepared to take the risk associated with HRT. I searched for the most well-informed specialists on the subject of bio-identical HRT and settled into a low-dose regime, which I still take today. This definitely helped with the levels of dryness, but good additional lubrication was still needed. Having had one particularly bad bout of soreness while using a new lubricant, which was so severe that my vulval skin was torn and bleeding, I decided to write to the manufacturer explaining my symptoms and ask for a list of ingredients. They replied saying that they took my complaint very seriously but could not tell me the ingredients, as it was commercially sensitive information. Finally the penny was beginning to drop. Maybe my symptoms for all these years had been as a result of the lubricant I was using. This might explain why the doctors had been unable to give me a full diagnosis other than say I had eczema.

In 2008 I discovered two women who had developed the world's first range of organic intimate lubricants, a pioneering new approach to intimate health. At this point, I had no idea that they would hold the key to unlocking the mystery of the long-lasting symptoms which had so affected my life. Their product, a certified organic intimate lubricant, is free of all petro-chemicals (as used in other lubricants), parabens (a preservative found in some breast tumours), glycerine (can be a mucosal irritant) and is formulated with natural plant-based gums. Having sensitive skin already, I was obviously reacting not only to the glycerine in lubricants but also to other harsh chemical ingredients.

The first time I used this organic product, I was amazed at how natural it felt and how it protected the sensitive tissue. I experienced no side effects, and at last, after almost 40 years, I was able to relax and know that intimacy and passion, still an important part of our marriage even in our early sixties, would not lead to days of soreness, irritation and discomfort. Painful sex is now a thing of the past.

I hope that telling my story will raise awareness of the importance of natural intimacy products, and help other women to realise that non-medical solutions may be part of the key to solving their intimate problems with painful sex too."

What do all of these changes mean? Well, as you've probably guessed by now, at the very least they'll change how you feel about yourself and your identity. That can be a good thing or a different thing. It might feel like a bad thing in the short term, but it doesn't have to be – and that's what I'm here to help with.

All of these changes might lead to difficult interactions and conversations in your relationship. You might feel you're growing distant from one another, or lack intimacy where you once were like sexed-up rabbits. At the far end of the scale, that lack of intimacy can be a contributing factor to marriage dissatisfaction and even divorce. John and Julie Gottman's 2011 study found that two thirds (67 per cent) of couples are reportedly less happy in their relationships after the arrival of a first baby,[11] which sums up nicely what I've been trying to say. This shit is hard. And you're not alone if you're struggling. BUT! There is also a lot you can do to help you and your relationship out of this hole, and that's what I want us to focus on.

Get Your Mojo Back 101

Dr Alexandra Kasozi, clinical psychotherapist, @the_psyched_mama

"We know that depression is linked to a reduced libido, and the same is true of postpartum depression, although it's harder to find research that deals with postpartum depression and libido specifically. Suffering from depression, and anxiety and trauma, can definitely make a difference to libido and stem interest in sex. In relation to the impact of PTSD on libido, one of the symptoms of post-traumatic distress is hyperarousal. When we are in a hyperaroused state, we are in a state of high alert and ready to respond to danger. We're producing more cortisol (the hormone produced in response to stress), and in those with PTSD, our brains are scanning our environment constantly for potential threats. Imagine that feeling of being on edge, highly anxious, easily startled, perhaps having an increased heart rate and struggling to relax. When we have been through trauma, and in particular when we have PTSD, we're stuck in that state. This is not a state that is conducive to relaxation or intimacy and sex.

Equally, if you've experienced a traumatic birth, you may also be suffering from very low mood or postnatal depression as well. You might be asking 'Am I normal? What's happening? Why am I not enjoying motherhood? Why aren't I feeling bonded and attached to my baby?' If you've experienced birth trauma, you're significantly more likely to also experience episodes or periods of depression and anxiety, even if they're not medically diagnosed. And all of these things, of course, can impact intimacy.

For example, it can also feel, when your partner touches you, that he wants something from you. And the baby wants something from you. And there are a million things that you're needed for. So the meaning of sex, and the meaning of your body and identity, can change – it's different to before. Your response might change from 'Oh, they want me!' to 'Ugh, they want me'. It can be hard to be needed all the time, and it can help to set some boundaries to spend time on your own to counter this."

What Next?

So now we know a bit more about what's happening in our bodies and why, let's look at what we can do to improve the situation.

1. **Take some time** (yes, I know it's bloody hard to find that time as a new parent) to really feel into which, if any, of these issues might be affecting you. What are your symptoms? What are you feeling? How does it trouble you? Can you make a note of any of this and start to make sense of it?
2. **Talk to your partner:** Or if you don't have a partner, try a supportive friend or family member. Just start with one thing that you want them to know. I know it's tough, especially when some of your feelings are hard for even you to understand – and articulating them is even tougher. But maybe even saying one sentence about how you're feeling will mean the rest flows more easily. Try these:
   a. "I feel XXX [eg odd, sad, awkward]."
   b. "My body feels XXX [eg unfamiliar, different] and I'm not sure how I feel about it."
   c. "I'm tired and I don't know what I'm doing."
   d. "Can you help me with XXX? [eg the washing, getting some nappies, making a bottle, booking my postnatal check-up or a massage] I'm finding it hard to find the time/energy."

As women, we are conditioned to think we can handle it all and it's our role to take care of everyone and everything. Letting someone know that that isn't the case isn't something we often do, but it's a simple step to make sure they know more about what you need. See Chapter 5 for more ways to talk to your partner and open up the conversation.

3. **Write it down:** Sometimes the words are just stuck in our throats. How about writing it down? You don't have to be eloquent or word-perfect, you don't have to have super neat handwriting or a pretty notebook; it doesn't even have to make much sense or be in proper sentences. But sometimes scribbling down the biggest thoughts and worries in your head can help you to be honest with yourself and to make sense of them. Clarity can come while you're writing them down (when you figure out how to write it down, those jumbled thoughts tend to unjumble), or they can act as a cathartic brain dump so that you can get it all out of your head (the relief!) and ponder it at a later date. Some call it journalling, or you can think of it as keeping a diary. But it doesn't have to have a name if that makes it feel like yet another thing on the to-do list, or something that isn't right for you. Just start. My favourite prompt sentence (write down the whole thing and then keep going) is "The biggest word in my head today is . . ." Once you've had a few goes at this, you might find it easier to express yourself verbally. Or you can also try writing a note to your partner and seeing how that opens things up for you both.

4. **Visit your GP** to ask for a referral. Can you figure out in advance which expert you might need to see? Though I hate to say it, make sure you're armed with the confidence and evidence to advocate for yourself, as it might not be straightforward. Do your research, too – I'm not saying read everything by Dr Google and believe it all, but do have a realistic think about which symptoms you are experiencing and their likely cause. Utterly bamboozled

and don't know where to start? Feel free to DM me on Insta @andbreathewellbeing.

5. **Look at therapy or visit a physio:** For me, it took a long time to acknowledge that I needed more help than I could give myself. I kept expecting things to get better by themselves, and that won't always work. I also struggled to acknowledge that it was okay to want and accept help. Accepting help doesn't mean you're broken; it actually means you're stronger than you were, and brave enough to realise what you need.

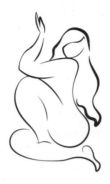

YOU WANT TO *WHAT?!*

Getting a handle on the gamut of physical symptoms.

We are often left bemused and disappointed by completely unexpected pain during penetrative sex after childbirth. It's not just one or two of us. Up to 83 per cent of us are experiencing dyspareunia (the medical term for painful sex) when we get intimate after giving birth.[1] Why is this? Why aren't we warned? Like so many things in women's health, our postnatal sex experience is not often talked about. We assume what we're experiencing is normal (rather than common); in the meantime, our pain is underplayed, while support is under-resourced. In this chapter I'll explain exactly how you can be affected by both caesarean and vaginal births and how you can start to find the answers.

At your six-week postnatal check-up – one of the only consistent, maternally focused touchpoints in the postnatal period the world over – where you might reasonably expect to discuss the issue, you'll usually be asked only about what contraception you'd like to go on to. In the UK, the NHS is a wonderful but very stretched service, and in other countries, such as the US, there are other healthcare system difficulties (such as cost) to contend with. Ask for a referral to a women's health physio, and you might have a fight on your hands, or your insurance company might not want to pay out. I've heard from some women whose GPs have genuinely been confused at the request and how it might help, and others whose doctors have questioned whether a problem is "serious" enough. I was equally clueless and didn't realise I was being passed from pillar to post until I finally discovered the reason for my issues over a year into my postnatal journey.

This chapter is about highlighting some of the pain you might feel, or equally the numbness you may experience – both can be equally worrying and discomfiting – discussing what's normal and what's common (they're not necessarily the same thing) and uncovering some of the causes of these symptoms. It's important to get clued up on these points, so that next time you go to your GP or other health professional, you can go armed with the right information, a set of questions to ask and the strength to advocate for yourself. Have a squizz at the Resources section at the end of the book for a free *Postnatal & Beyond Wellbeing Checklist* that you can take with you to your six-to-eight-week appointment with the GP, or any other medical appointment.

No matter how you gave birth – at home or hospital, in water or on dry land, whether you called them surges or contractions, and whether your baby made a vaginal or caesarean entrance to the world – the amazing work of our bodies to create, grow and birth a baby is intense. For vaginal births, the uterus, pelvic floor and vaginal canal literally transform themselves to bring new life into the world. The work that our bodies do after caesareans to recover from major abdominal surgery, all with a demanding baby to feed and sleepless nights to get through, is incredible.

If you were scared, unprepared or worried about childbirth and gave birth vaginally, your body (and mind) may have experienced some trauma or bruising. If you were comfortable, joyful and at one with giving birth, your uterus still expanded to *over 100 times its empty size*[2] to fit a baby – that's a momentous event in itself!

The cervix dilates from completely closed (the opening just a little dimple on its surface) to at least 10cm (4in) wide[3] to fit a baby's head and then body through it. The distance that the uterus, cervix and pelvic floor flex and stretch is utterly mind-blowing, incredible work. The fact that your body knows how to do this is primeval and amazing. But it can also be a tad uncomfortable.

For example, from a physiological point of view, when you are fearful, your body can go into fight or flight mode, blocking feel-good hormones like oxytocin. Oxytocin is needed to help relax and flex the muscles in your uterus and cervix, and these movements help get the baby out through your vagina. Without enough oxytocin to ease and encourage the journey, your fear ends up pitting your body against, well, your body.

So whether you found your body suited or not to vaginal childbirth, it's an incredible (in the true sense of the word) experience. One for which you can give yourself a gigantic pat on the back.

If you gave birth abdominally by caesarean, this required cutting through seven layers of skin, tissue and muscle. It's not the easy option, though you may have heard people say it is. A C-section is major abdominal surgery, and while it can be beautiful, healing and gentle if planned, it may also be traumatic if unplanned. Unplanned caesareans, or what we often refer to as "emergency" C-sections, from Category 1 (immediate threat to life) to Category 3 (unplanned), account for around half of caesareans in the UK[4] – so they are relatively common, but the aftercare advice can be surprisingly scant. How you feel coming out of your C-section birth, how you heal and how you process the experience in the longer term can all be affected by how you felt about it to begin with.

We often think that it's only vaginal births that can have a detrimental effect on our pelvic floor. So when pain, numbness or painful sex are part of our postnatal journey, it can be confusing and worrying. But whatever form your birth took, you'll have some level of trauma to your body for which you need, and deserve, time to heal.

The Start of My Postnatal Journey

A while after giving birth, I started to deal with the sexual pain I was experiencing, speaking about it more, doing research and seeking advice. As I did so, the realisation dawned that what I was experiencing was common, and worryingly so. It was often spoken about and thought of as normal, shrugged off by sufferers as something that happens postnatally (along with things like wetting yourself after you've had a baby, more on which later too) and glossed over by medical professionals in the rehabilitation journey.

The more I experience, and the more I work in this field, the more I believe sexual dysfunction after birth (or any rehabilitation issues postnatally) shouldn't be common, and we should not accept it as normal. The first person I turned to for help, my GP, who referred me to gynaecologists at the hospital, was unhelpful. But I didn't know who to ask for further advice or what to do instead. Ultimately, these difficulties led to the discovery of who *could* help, and taught me who I could or should have turned to in the first place and how important it is to know my own body and be able to advocate for myself.

Here's what happened to me to get me started on that journey – how the birth impacted me mentally and physically and how I started to recognise that something wasn't right.

My Story

Now I had a baby. Despite (or perhaps because of) those long months we'd spent waiting for (or denying the reality of) her arrival, it was a shock to the system to have her screaming in our arms once we actually got there.

We spent two days in hospital, in a daze from the birth, in a room with a cot but no baby. Our daughter was in NICU for four days. Bryn bedded down on the floor on a camping mattress. I was syringing colostrum[5] from my recalcitrant, aching boobs to take to the ward to feed Delphi, supplementing the bottles she was being given. When I was discharged after two days, Delphi stayed in for another two, so we left hospital without her. I don't think I registered it at the time, but when I think of that moment now, I feel a wrench.

So we spent those two days going back and forth between hospital and home. I remember with muffled clarity the first awful night that we had her at home. I was dizzy with tiredness because I didn't know how to settle her, what to do next, what her cries meant, why I couldn't get her to stop. The night was so, so long, and I was so lost.

Daylight came, the days and weeks passed, and we muddled through. Always two steps forward and one and a half back. This new human didn't do what all the books said it should, damn it. I floundered in my unknowingness. My postnatal depression crept into my brain and squatted like an unwelcome visitor. My stress reaction to the birth trauma was a surprise too. I don't think I knew that birth trauma could be a thing, but I couldn't get it out of my head; I re-lived it, almost enjoying the nightmares, like when you keep picking at a scab despite knowing it's making it worse. I didn't realise until a few years later that this was a trauma reaction, because I was so busy and worried anyway that I couldn't allow myself to think about how I was (or wasn't) processing the birth.

So what could I do but carry on? I focused on controlling what I could and got angry when I couldn't. The postpartum rage (I didn't know at the time that it was called that) was yet another thing I hadn't been prepared for. For me it was an expression of postnatal depression, but, with the clarity that you get from having been through it, it's also totally understandable for any new parents, given the stress and sleep deprivation we're under. But when it was happening, in that truly confusing time, it felt horrible and wrong, and like I wasn't being the mother I was supposed to be.

I felt like a failure because I didn't know what I was doing, the baby didn't do what she was supposed to and my body, it was turning out, didn't take to motherhood like I thought it would either. Because I'd been away from my baby for four days, I hadn't been able to breastfeed. I expressed, but my breasts just wouldn't produce milk for a machine. I remember a midwife passing by and saying, "You've been going for 30 minutes – you should have much more milk than that by now." I looked accusingly at the tiny dribble of milk in the bottom of the bottle, but I couldn't do anything about it. The more I pumped, the more tense I became, so that even if my boobs had known how to let down without a baby on them, it would have been a futile exercise.

With hindsight I know that that small amount would have been enough. Babies have teeny tiny stomachs when they are first born. Plus some boobs, like mine, just don't respond well to breast pumps. Oh no, they only let down for a proper baby, thank you very much – even once breastfeeding was established, it was impossible to express any meaningful amount of milk for bottles, and it's been the same with my second baby too.

But at the time, while I was trying to stimulate them, like a failing cow, and feeling increasingly worse about myself, it only added to the overall emotional burden I was gathering. Once we'd left hospital, we soldiered on. Through the tongue-tie (her), screaming hunger (her and me), pain (me) and blood blisters on nipples (definitely me), a mere three weeks later, we'd cracked it. It was touch and go, not just for the breastfeeding, but for my sanity at times, and though three weeks doesn't sound like a lot, when you have a piranha clamping on one of the most sensitive parts of your body several times a day and through the night, three weeks feels like a lifetime. It was only my stubbornness that got us through it, but I know that I was horrible to be around at the time, and I felt horrible in myself. I don't know, actually, whether it was worth it in the end, when I think about the build-up of guilt and shame and the long-lasting impact that it had on my mental health.

Then there was my body. I had put on weight during the pregnancy and was (or told everyone I was) fine with that, knowing I'd lose it in time. In actual fact, I was nervous. Who wouldn't be at such a momentous transformation of the body that's carried you for your whole life? Things that I could feel positive about: my tummy muscles were always strong, so with breathing and core engagement exercises, my bump went down smoothly and quickly. My skin had stretched without any tiger stripes, and was still soft and supple; I used to moisturise it every day as a thank you for its service. I felt at least like this was something that was going right, that I could control.

When I read this back, when I think about my battered self at that time, I ask myself why this, my body, was the positive thing that I grasped for. Why was it that the only thing that I felt I was doing well at, that made me feel good, was the very thing that meant I would be conforming to type? It wasn't the fact that we'd made it through another day with a newborn, or marvelling at the miracle of life that my husband and I had created. Instead I was feeling secretly smug that my tummy was disappearing, like it should. I shouldn't, after all, want to look like I'd had a baby, should I?! I didn't *not* feel awe at the baby, but it was definitely muted. I more distinctly remember how I felt about myself during that time. There's also a lot of time, energy, words and art dedicated to that miracle of new life. There's less space given over to us as the bearers of new life, and how we cope, body and mind. So that's what I want to focus on and normalise.

However, despite my smugness, my body did have something else in store for me. It's never a straight road, is it? During my pregnancy I'd been obsessed with doing my pelvic floor exercises. I was determined they would not succumb to post-birth weakness. I would keep a strong pelvic floor if it killed me! After birth, I felt the same. Along with the breathing and core engagement, it was the one thing I felt confident of, having been a keen and confident fitness person for all of my adult life. My pelvic floor exercises had become a habit, almost an inadvertent tic, as I did them so much. Squeeze, squeeze, squeeze. As hard as you can! Stronger! Longer! I was determined that this was something that I would get right. However, one thing that I never did properly, because I didn't know I should be, was release the lift. When you tense a muscle, any muscle, to train it, you also need to release it afterwards properly; otherwise, it might become big, but it won't be much use functionally. I didn't know this, and because I was only interested in building the muscle to be as strong as it could be, it didn't occur to me to ask either.

It was telling that Kegels were the thing I obsessed over, when I could, and perhaps should, have been focused on my all-round recovery and my baby's health. I ended up with a hypertonic[6] (too tight) pelvic floor, which I would only discover 13 months after I'd given birth, along with the super-sensitive scars which went alongside it.

The focus on my body was, I think, because I wanted to prove that I was fine and ready to be me again. I wanted to feel more like my pre-baby self. I longed to feel unencumbered and at ease in my body and mind. I ached to feel confident and, yes, sexy and sexual. I didn't understand where I had gone as a person. I was technically still me, but I wasn't. I was a mother, and I didn't know how this slotted into me. It was all so new and odd. Some people find this transition an easy one to make, but I didn't.

In a bid to feel more like me, I decided that I wanted to have sex again. Six weeks postnatally, it seemed like a good time to try it. After the check-up with my GP (yes, we had the contraceptive chat, it was about the only thing that I was asked about myself) and in the living room so as not to disturb the baby, we attempted our first bout of intimacy as parents. Having had a second baby now, I don't know how on earth I had the energy, but the fact that I wanted to push through, with no thought to my actual wellbeing, shows how discombobulated I was feeling.

Of course Bryn was willing, but I was the instigator. He was led by my surface-level enthusiasm. And how do you say no to a slightly manic new mother anyway? I can tell you now that I wouldn't have reacted kindly! When it came to it, it wasn't the right thing to do. The sex was so painful it was like shards of broken glass in my vagina. The wrong-headed part of me wanted to carry on – despite feeling, knowing, that something was wrong. Perhaps if we tried a little longer, the pain would ease. But it didn't. I was in tears because I was in so much pain, but also because I felt I had let both myself and my husband down. Things were yet again not going as expected, and I didn't know why or how to fix it.

Of course we stopped. And I licked my wounds. We cuddled and talked, and ultimately the experience prompted me to identify all of the things that were wrong that I hadn't even heard of before. But that would take many months, and I would be too scared to try to have sex again for a long time. I've mentioned my hypertonic pelvic floor muscles already, which are more common than you'd think, but I also suffered from a lack of lubrication, and the sensitive vaginal scar tissue that I've also talked about. Added to this are the only-to-be-expected-with-a-vaginal-birth vulvodynia (sensitivity of the vulva around the vaginal opening) and, of course, tension, which I experienced as a reaction to the trauma of the birth and a wariness of penetration, which is pretty obvious when you think about it, but which I barely countenanced as a possibility. I figured that everyone else went through things like this, so why should I be the only one to have a problem with it afterwards? I'm not the only one, of course; I just thought I was, because we don't talk about these things.

Scars and Stripes: How Your Body Might Change

There are a myriad of ways you could be feeling in your vagina and abdomen. We've talked about how much pregnancy and childbirth changes your body, and we know that it doesn't recover immediately. Neither do your feelings. Processing the monumental fact of childbirth, particularly if it's your first birth, also takes time. We'll come back to the mind later, but first let's tackle the more pressing problem of physical pain, particularly when it's triggered by unusual positions, such as sex or penetration.

If you're feeling a bit run-through-the-mill by the miracle of life, it could be caused by a number of things and will take different amounts of time to heal depending on the cause of the pain and the person. Figuring all of this out can be like untangling a ball of string. Hopefully you'll find the end of your thread here so you can figure out what might be behind the symptoms, but please always visit a health professional (such as your GP, gynaecologist or women's health physio) to get your in-depth questions answered.

Bear in mind that it's completely normal to experience mild to medium pains, aches or lack of sensation in either your pelvic floor, vagina or abdomen . . . but it's not normal for it to be severe, or for it to last. So if you are feeling lots of pain for a long period of time, this could be a sign of something more serious, and it's a good idea to see your doctor.

Sharp Pain

Yikes! Uncomfortable is not the word. And unfortunately all too many women are experiencing sharp pain during sex postnatally. This could be due to a few different reasons, so let's visit number one on the list.

Wounds and Scars

It's not unusual to have a wound, bruising or scarring inside the vagina or in the vulval area; these can be of varying degrees and caused by various processes. Even the most peaceful of births involves a human being squeezing out of your vagina, which is not a gentle process.

An episiotomy (also known as perineotomy) is a cut between the vaginal and anal openings, usually off to one side to avoid a fourth-degree tear running directly between the vagina and anus. Episiotomies might seem the obvious reason for scarring on the vaginal tissue – because it's the only time you're cut down there.

In actual fact, you may have grazing, tears or small cuts inside the vagina itself from the delivery of the baby, with or without intervention. If your baby birthed without intervention, the likelihood of tearing or grazing is much smaller, but if you experienced a suction/ventouse or forceps delivery, the chances of grazing on your vaginal walls are much higher due to the insertion of instruments.

But why does it *still* hurt? Imagine a paper cut on your finger. It's tiny but it stings like hell. Now imagine a cut or graze inside your vagina. Perhaps you just winced a little. I did. As women, we have a tendency to play down our cuts and scrapes, suck it up and get on with it. Especially when it comes to such a natural process as childbirth.

Small cuts hurt more than you think. One that stings mildly when you're upright and walking about will be hugely aggravated when it experiences the friction of penetrative sex. If you have a larger graze or tear, the pain may be correspondingly bigger.

If you've had a caesarean birth, your scar is the biggest, most obvious wound of all! Here we're dealing with surgical incisions to several layers of tissue, not just the surface wound, so it can take at least six to twelve weeks to heal, though all our bodies are different. The surface wound will probably heal faster, but you may experience discomfort and pain internally, particularly during your period and as a result of any other internal workings, including penetrative sex. The scar itself is significant (though I promise it will look much better in a few months!) and that surface and internal scar tissue can have an impact on your other core muscles, like your abdominal muscles, pelvic floor and even the muscles around your hips and thighs. If you missed it, I talked a lot more about how to care for and massage your scar in Chapter 2.

Bruising

Even without any abrasions, bruising can also cause pain. Imagine you've done a super hardcore workout. Your muscles can ache for days afterwards if you move them in a certain way, stress them by repeating the workout movements or even poke them inadvertently. Now transfer that image to your vaginal and uterine muscles, and any pain you're feeling might make a little more sense.

And sorry to be the bearer of bad news, but once any wound has healed, the pain doesn't necessarily go away. Scars are formed of newly created tissue, and so haven't had time to toughen up like the rest of your skin. Often scar tissue is also raised, so the new, sensitive tissue sits proud of the surface and is more likely to be touched or irritated. Both these factors mean that scars are usually incredibly sensitive, so whereas touching a scar on the surface of the body might induce a shiver, for a scar inside your vagina this sensitivity is ramped up to pain. For the worst cases, you may experience pain while walking or sitting (that blow-up hemorrhoid ring never looked so good!), and again, the friction of penetrative sex will act directly on any scars you might have. In the worst cases, pain may feel searing, but if this is you, don't be alarmed – the likelihood is that we can help get you back to where you want to be.

But We Can't See It!

The little problem with your sex organs, if you're a biological woman, is that you can't see these miraculous parts of your body. This is a bit of a disadvantage when we're trying to get to grips with them as a teenager, let alone understanding what role they have in defining us as grown-ups, then as new mums and later as we enter perimenopause.

The imagery that we are presented with to understand our sex organs is either purely scientific or uniquely over-sexualised, such as in the cartoon-like cross-sections of the body in school biology textbooks or in the proliferation of waxed pussies in male-gaze-led porn.

These images are almost all white – in fact I saw the first black reproductive diagram in 2021. Most of us have trouble finding a comfortable middle ground (whatever that might be for you) in between these two contrasting ends of the scale, let alone an image that is relatable.

So here are a couple more helpful renderings of your body. From the different angles, you can now understand more about how big the pelvic floor is (so no wonder it causes a lot of problems if you're lacking strength there); how small the uterus is when empty and how large it can get with a baby inside; and how squished your organs all get when you're pregnant, and so how far they have to travel to slot back into place afterwards.

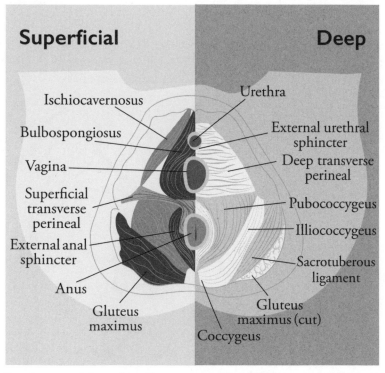

Rendering of the pelvic floor as seen from below.

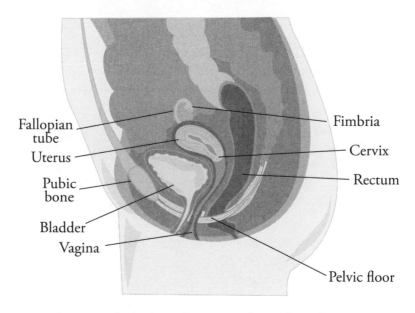

Internal organs of a biological woman, shown from the upper thighs to the mid-abdomen (not pregnant).

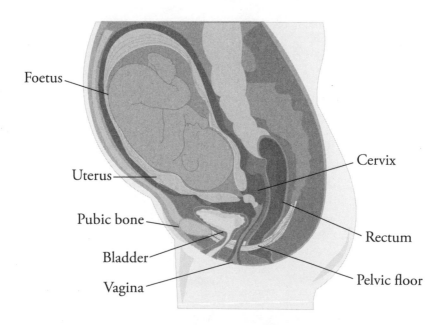

Internal organs of a biological woman (pregnant).

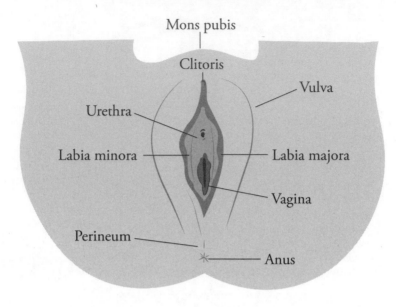

Diagram of the vulval area before a vaginal birth.

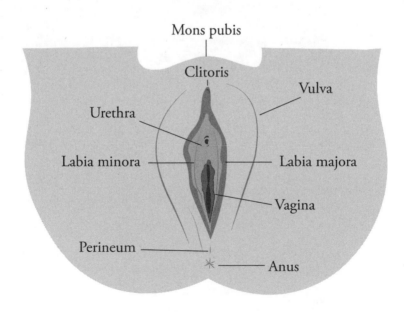

The vulval area after a vaginal birth: note the smaller perineal gap.

Take a Peek

A useful exercise, if you haven't done it already (or even if you have!), is to take a mirror, or your cellphone/mobile, and spend some time looking at your own vulva. Don't feel embarrassed about it – men have an obsession with their penises, so why shouldn't we have a peek at vulvas? It's time to normalise the vulva and our own sexuality.

It might feel weird the first time you do – that's only normal for something we usually ignore – but the longer you look at it, and if you do it regularly, the more comfortable you'll get. This is especially important to do post-childbirth, particularly if you had a vaginal birth.

Our vaginas and vulvas are stretched and change through the process of birth. Getting to grips with what yours looks like, or what it looks like *now*, is a really important part of knowing yourself and understanding how your body works and feels. If you are experiencing any differences with intimacy and sex, this is especially important. Knowing yourself physically will help identify the causes of any issues or worries.

If you have struggled with your experience of birth (whatever that looks like for you), looking at your vulva – indeed, even opening your legs at all! – can also be quite an emotional thing to do. Amanda Savage, my favourite women's health physio, told me that she often spends time with women in postnatal consultations simply being present with them at the top end of their bodies while they adjust to the feeling of butterflying their legs and feeling the air on their vulva. It can bring back a rush of feelings, and it's important to give time to these to enable yourself to process them.

Vaginal Sensitivity

Even if you don't have any wounds, scarring or bruising, your vagina may be feeling more sensitive than normal. It might not sound like a big deal, but when we're talking about penetrative sex (if that's your aim), sensitivity can quickly tip over into pain.

This sensitivity can be called vaginitis or vulvodynia, depending on where it is, and how long it lasts. You may experience redness, irritation and dryness in your vagina or vulva area. Though both are without an exact cause, after childbirth these conditions can be exacerbated by banal things like your usual laundry detergent, sitting in a funny position, birth injuries or bruising, imbalanced or weakened pelvic floor muscles and the biggie: changes in hormonal levels.

Those damned hormone ebbs and flows can cause one huge change that we often don't expect: a lack of vaginal lubrication. For example, breastfeeding means more prolactin and oxytocin in the body, but it also lowers your oestrogen levels for as long as you're nursing. Oestrogen is responsible for lubrication throughout the body, so it's no wonder it has an impact on your vaginal tissues too. As if we didn't have enough to deal with.

This lack of lubrication coupled with irritable tissue can be incredibly painful – I should know! Hormone balance can be tweaked and improved in the longer term, but reducing stress levels, getting your nutrition right and sleeping a full night are probably not too easy in the first few months or years of motherhood. So don't be afraid, in the early days and beyond, to reach for the lube. While we tend to think of it as taboo, there's really nothing to be wary of, and it can make things a whole lot more fun. Read more about vaginal lubricants later in this chapter and in Chapter 7 (and throughout this book, frankly: I love lube).

Get Your Mojo Back 101

Lavinia Winch – women's health champion and lube expert

"An organic lubricant must contain a very high percentage of natural ingredients and be free from harmful chemicals or additives. The organic certification provides transparency about the ingredients, their source and the business and manufacturing processes of the brand. The company and the laboratory are audited annually by an accrediting body such as the Soil Association. Some products will claim that they are 'natural', but this is not the same as being 'Certified Organic'.

Equally important is the formulation of the lubricant because the vaginal environment is finely balanced and protected by the vaginal flora or microbiome. A healthy vaginal flora protects the body against urogenital infections such as UTIs, thrush and bacterial vaginosis. It is made up of many different types of probiotic bacteria, the predominant bacteria being lactobacilli. Indeed, these lactobacilli and candida species often co-exist in the vagina of healthy women. Lactobacilli protect against vaginal infection simply by colonising the space available. They build up a barrier against candidal overgrowth by blocking the adhesion of candidal yeast cells to vaginal epithelial cells, through competition for nutrients. They also produce lactic acid and hydrogen peroxide. Lactic acid helps to maintain a healthy vaginal pH and flora. Hydrogen peroxide stops the overgrowth of 'bad' bacteria that cause infection. When the level of lactobacilli is disrupted and the vaginal flora becomes imbalanced, the risk of developing an infection is increased. The infections can lead to unpleasant symptoms such as itching, irritation, burning, abnormal discharge and unpleasant vaginal odour.

The balance between beneficial and harmful bacteria in the vagina is very fragile, and an imbalance occurs if the vaginal pH is not acidic enough. The vaginal pH should be somewhere between 3.8 and 4.5 for a healthy level of vaginal acidity. If the vagina is not acidic enough due to a shortage of lactobacilli, then fungi and 'bad' bacteria are able to reproduce more than they usually would. This crucial balance can be easily disrupted by ingredients that change the vaginal pH, so all lubricants should clearly state the pH on the pack. Ingredients that can easily irritate the vagina or disrupt the fragile flora include glycerine, glycols, perfume and flavourings such as might be found in non-organic product."

Dull Ache

Think of your body as like a house. During pregnancy your insides were rejigged like the rooms of the house being reshuffled. The bathroom is where the living room was, the bedrooms are in the kitchen and the utility room's been relegated to the garden. It's a hell of a lot to go through, and it's only to be expected that it takes a bit of work to get them back to where you want them to be.

Plus, midwives and obstetricians or surgeons and nurses have been rummaging around in your insides. Muscles have been stretched and they're only just thinking about shrinking back to their previous size. So it should come as no surprise that you might not be feeling quite as tip-top as you were before pregnancy.

While we might expect (or feel pressure for) our bodies to snap back to pre-pregnancy form, you've been through a lot, and it will take time for those changes to right themselves. A bit, or a lot, of cramping can be normal as your uterus begins to shrink back to its empty size, particularly if you're breastfeeding, as this prompts the body's contraction response. Though a lot of shrinking happens in the hours and days post-birth, you'll be seeing and feeling changes even in the weeks and months after your baby arrives. And during all this time, you might be feeling a tad tender.

Give yourself a break, and if you're feeling achy during sex and it's not for you right now, let your partner know and back off the sexy times a little.

Digging Pain

Heads up: your cervix, miracle that your body is, moves up and down during your cycle to make it easier or harder for sperm to reach the uterus. I know, right? Our bodies are incredible. But also, as part of the internal house renovations that your body goes through with pregnancy and birth, after birth your uterus and cervix might be sitting in a slightly different place.

When the cervix sits low, any kind of penetrative sex can be uncomfortable for some couples, depending on how low your cervix sits and the size of your frame. This can cause an uncomfortable poking, pushing and bruising sensation for some women at different times in their cycle, and it might be worse after childbirth as your body and your cycle shifts back to where it should be. So if it's not comfortable for you, stop. Try again at a different time. There's no rush to get back in the sack if you're not ready.

No Feeling

But what if there's no feeling at all? The absence of sensation can be just as emotionally taxing as pain itself. Perhaps it's even worse, because it ties in with societal dialogue around loose vaginas and the complete absence of sexual pleasure once you've had a baby.

Stop! Please don't be disheartened. I wouldn't leave you there, and this doesn't mean the end of the coital road. After all, most people go on to have second (and more) children, don't they? Despite single-child families being the fastest-growing category of household set-up, they still make up only around 20 per cent of families.[7] But let's make this about more than just lying back and thinking of your favourite ice cream flavour.

The nerves in your vagina are sensitive things, and they have probably been bruised by a baby descending through the birth canal – it's a tight fit, you know. Some of the nerve endings as well as the surrounding tissue might be bruised, and in nerves, bruising means numbness or tingliness, rather than the sensations you're used to.

As with everything I've been talking about, it can take a while for sensation to come back to these nerves, so don't pull the emergency cord just yet. It takes different amounts of time for different people, but if you're still experiencing numbness at your six-week check-up after the birth, make sure to mention it to your GP and seek further advice.

As we've touched on previously, whatever you are feeling (or not) in your vagina can also be affected by any wound healing and the strength/weakness and flexibility of your pelvic floor. So, say it with me now: it's a good idea to get physically examined internally by a women's health physiotherapist to check your muscles are working properly and whether you're doing your pelvic floor lifts effectively.

Bear in mind that the vaginal walls are pretty elastic, and the vagina is designed to do exactly the right amount of stretching and shrinking back after childbirth. If you feel that you don't have enough sensation or that things are a little loose, they usually improve a lot in the first few weeks post-birth. So if you're trying out nooky early in your postnatal journey, it might be worth waiting a couple more months and monitoring any improvement that happens naturally. Once that's happened and you feel there's further to go for you to get the pleasure you deserve, there are plenty of avenues to explore.

Get Your Mojo Back 101

Amanda Savage – women's health physiotherapist
@propelvic

"Our nerves run in a two-way system. Sensations come up to the brain from the pelvic floor. In the immediate aftermath of delivery, this system can be poor. If sensations are not coming up, then they're likely not going down either. Your muscles won't be reacting to brain signals. If muscles aren't reacting, they sit floppy. This makes the vagina feel gaping or bigger. Mums talk about feeling loose or big, open or weak. You might not like sex because you're not getting any pleasure out of it. Naturally, you're also concerned that your partner's not getting the feelings they want either, and that can be what most women think is going to happen when they have a baby. This lack of sensation can be caused by scarring too, because the scar tissue can be numb for a while.

Mums say they feel like they have 'weak' muscles. But it's important to explore whether the muscles are *truly* weak; perhaps instead they are not working? 'Weak' and 'not working' are not quite the same thing. A weak muscle would be one that has had a long period of not being used, say because you were carrying the weight of twins or it was a very big baby. You maybe didn't pay much attention to the pelvic floor when you were pregnant and then it got a big stretch. In which case it's going to take quite a long time to come back from a place of true weakness. Just like if your leg got weak because you were in a plaster for six weeks, it's going to take quite a while to build strength back up.

But sometimes the pelvic floor is what we call inhibited. You've literally had such a shock to the system, your brain can't remember what to do with your muscles. Physios see this issue sometimes with footballers who come in to have a camera put in their knee, and then they can't get up and walk. The shock of it makes their muscles that are perfectly alright 'forget' how to work.

Mums can recover fast from this inhibited/weak place because they just need to get their head and their muscles reconnected. They'll see improvement in a couple of weeks. Or you might have a *true* weakness where you've literally got to wait for that muscle to build itself up over the course of months. This is why mums have such different experiences post-baby.

For example, nerve damage can also be a factor: pudendal nerve latency. Up to six months after the birth, you can find poor neural flow through the pudendal nerve that supplies the pelvic floor.[8] This is a physiological problem. Messages are only very slowly making their way to your pelvic floor, so by the time you need the pelvic floor to have moved, it's too late, which can cause leaks.

It's often also a mental health issue. So many times I'll say to a mum: 'Do you think you've switched off below the belly button as a way of coping with what you just went through?' Many times delivery has been a traumatic experience – maybe not 'officially', but on a personal emotional level. It's a big experience, to expose all your private parts to an awful lot of people! Mums don't realise how vulnerable they can feel until they've been through it, and they often don't process everything until afterwards. Perhaps there were too many people invading your private space, or maybe you were sent home scared and without guidance – the last memories you have of that space [your vagina and vulva] are not happy ones, so you just would rather not think about it.

Often what I'm trying to do as a physiotherapist is work out: do you need to do classic pelvic floor strength exercises? Or do we need to spend time reconnecting with your breathing, being aware that when you breathe you can feel your pelvic floor and how to relax it? Or do you need to be vulnerable in a space with a physio, revisiting things that you haven't yet wanted to or had time to, but need to? This could also be done with a psychologist or a counsellor, but often it is your physio who will offer that space to be vulnerable. Many of my patients find themselves crying, but I think we need to go through these steps in order to process our experience and help the brain allow the muscles to work again.

We should also talk about scarring. In contrast to the numbness – the not feeling enough – other mums feel too much, or experience pain, because scars themselves can be hypersensitive. You can't predict what kind of scars your body will make. There's also a difference between a tear and a cut. The best outcomes are when cuts or tears are stitched under lights [i.e. in theatre] by the most senior person present. Surprisingly, even minor grazes can be very sore too.

Your recovery is affected partly by the actual abrasion of the skin and the surface layers, which you can see or touch, but also by your body's reaction to that. If you hurt your hand, you know that your hand will close in on itself. You will protect it by holding it tense. The same can be true of pelvic floor injuries. We tense up to guard and protect them. A tense or guarding pelvic floor is termed 'hypertonic'.

We now know that scars in the abdomen (like caesarean scars) can have an influence on the pelvic floor too. Think of how a twist in a tee-shirt pulls fabric from further away toward it. Abdominal scars can change the position of the hips, legs and feet, usually turning them inward.

As penetrative sex is actually about getting your hips *out*, you need to be surprisingly mobile in your hips and pelvic joints to have good sex or to enjoy a variety of sexual positions. Good sex is not just about the tissues of the vagina. If your caesarean scar is pulling your hips toward each other, then opening your legs will be uncomfortable.

The passing of time can itself cause complications. If the postnatal body is left alone for a while before problems are addressed, I often describe it as like a child that's been learning to knit. They've been working by themselves and they've made errors and tried to fix them, but row by row they are making it worse. Finally they just hand you this jumbled mess of wool! To fix it, you've just got to start somewhere by unpicking a corner. For your postnatal body, picking at the easy wins is key. So I say 'let's start with lubricant', 'let's talk about processing trauma', 'let's start stretching the muscles around the pelvis'. These things help most mums. Once you start unpicking, some of the problem layers fall away really quickly.

Women (and society at large) often have preconceived ideas of what a body should be like after a baby. We know in our hearts that you can't grow a baby and deliver it, and expect this to have no physical impact on our life. Yet some mums are genuinely in shock that their body is different. Also, many women don't realise that they have to put any effort in to rehabilitate. Social media can make women believe that everybody else has just 'bounced back', and they want fixing because they haven't. They don't realise that others might have put a lot of work in, or are very lucky genetically.

It's good to both let go a bit and accept that life is different, and also accept that there's work to do. The mums that cope best, I've found, are the ones who can adapt. Darwin said, 'It is not the strongest of the species that survives, nor the most intelligent; it is the one most adaptable to change.' And that's particularly pertinent for entering motherhood, I think."

What Next?

Here are some practical things you can do to help, people you can ask, referrals you can seek and exercises you can do:

- Ask your GP to rule out infection.
- Ask to be referred to a women's health physio once this has been done if there's no improvement.
- Visit a women's health physio privately if you aren't referred and can afford it.
- Ascertain if you have any scarring, bruising, grazing and work out an action plan with your physio to desensitise and heal tissue and strengthen or relax your pelvic floor.
- Work out the source of your numbness or loose feeling and create an action plan to bring back sensation and/or strengthen your pelvic floor.
- Study your own vulva, the external part between your legs and around your vaginal opening, with a mirror (or take a picture on your cellphone/mobile!) and familiarise yourself with it. If you have any scars, you may be able to see these and understand them more intimately. The shape of your vagina may have changed too; this is completely normal.
- Gently check your vagina (the internal part) with your fingers. Wash your hands first, of course, and use lubrication if necessary, to test out the sensitivity of the different parts of your vaginal wall and the opening of the vagina.
- Start doing or continue to do your pelvic floor exercises, but make sure you're doing them properly (see page 47 onward for more).
- Have confidence: You're not alone, and whatever your experience, it can usually be vastly improved.
- Buy some lubricant! Lube is nothing to be ashamed of, and it will definitely make things a lot more comfortable and, hopefully, more pleasurable. If it doesn't, it's a really easy thing to have ticked off the list. Always go for an organic product; my favourite, and in my view the best, is YES Organics.

The Professionals

Unsure who might be your knight(ess) in shining armour? Here are a few of the most common medical and health professionals who could provide some more answers.

General Practitioner (GP): A doctor, usually the first port of call for medical advice in the NHS in the UK. You should usually be able to access a GP for free, especially if you have a young baby. In the US, doctor's visits, even for the baby, are not free but are usually covered by your insurance plan.

Women's Health Physiotherapist (UK) / Women's Health Physical Therapist (US): A physiotherapist/physical therapist specialising in women's bodies, especially through changes like pregnancy, childbirth/postnatal and the menopause. Has expert knowledge in pelvic floor and core health, and often birth trauma as well.

Gynaecologist: Specialist doctors focusing on women's health, in particular the reproductive system. They can deal with a wide range of issues such as fertility, pregnancy/childbirth, hormone imbalance, recurrent STIs, cancer, etc.

Pre/postnatal Personal Trainer: A specialist fitness instructor focusing on one-to-one training (rather than a group fitness instructor). Make sure the one you use is postnatally trained and experienced so that you are rehabilitated properly and pushed appropriately.

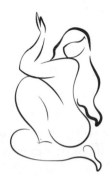

HOW ABOUT AFTER THE WASHING UP, DARLING?

Navigating the practicalities of intimacy in real life.

It might be a long journey, but once you're past the pain and identity shift, there's the more banal question of when to find the bloody time. We all joke about it, but let's be honest, the tiredness is REAL.

We're juggling sleepless nights, we're talking about sexy things like weaning, buying nappies, school drop-offs and work meetings. We're often stressed and trying to manage the shopping, the in-laws and our (haha) social lives all at once, too. Which all means that getting in the mood isn't quite as straightforward as it was pre-kids. This chapter explains why this is okay (surprise, surprise, it's not just you), and how to make things better and more enjoyable for you both. Because while it doesn't feel like it now, I promise you, it can get better and, dare I say it, easier.

Traditionally we've hidden how tricky parenthood can be, largely because the load has been carried by women, or subsumed by the "village" (friends and family, a support network that lives near you), or taken on by paid helpers and staff. Now, thank goodness, women are able to work more (huzzah!) and hold more responsibility in their careers and public life, and so the paid or unpaid work of trying to run a family and keep your kids alive is once again up for grabs. While we're trying to live more equally, the burden is still often carried by women, just as it always has been. It takes a lot to break this kind of convention.

I'm not advocating this, and I would love you to find ways to navigate it in your household setting, but even in the most equal of families, you realise that it's easier said than done to find time and headspace for you, your relationship and your sexuality. What's the first thing that gets dropped when we're busy? Usually for parents, and, dare I say it, even more so for mums, it's looking after yourself. With my wellbeing advocacy hat on, I bang on about self-care all the time. It's a concept that I hope we're familiar with now; we talk about it constantly. But when I first had my daughter, it was a newish concept, or at least a concept that was only just starting to get the airtime it deserves. We take it for granted now – people even mock it. But time for "you" is really vital to long-term happiness. And that doesn't just mean nipping to the nail salon once in a while: it means making sure you're getting the nourishment you need for body, mind and, yes, libido – once you've dug it out from under that pile of washing.

Esther Perel, whose brilliant work as a psychotherapist focuses on relationships and sexuality, says "many women tell me they're animated by being the turn on. Her flicker comes from inside, not from the other, and if she is not into it, nothing will happen. The unspoken truth about women's sexuality is how narcissistic it can be – in the best of ways. The female's ability to focus on herself is the pathway to erotic pleasure." Which is all very well, but what happens when we aren't able to find that focus? Focus is about time, space and the ability to guide your senses and your mind to one thing. That's not easy when you have to-do lists exploding out of drawers, and one ear's always on the baby monitor.

I love that Esther owns how narcissistic we as women can be, and indeed need to be, in the pursuit of sensuality and sexual pleasure. But motherhood is traditionally about being as un-narcissistic as possible. How do we marry those two ideas in the real world? And how do we make this work for us and our partners on a practical level? How on earth are we going to find time to have amazing sex again?!

Getting our Rhythm Back

The pain that I experienced on top of the identity issues I felt, both physically and mentally, led to a complete lack of confidence in myself and my body. I'd always been able to rely on it before, and it felt to me like it was now letting me down at every turn. I had to work hard to recalibrate. Sex was almost a non-issue because it had been so long since I'd thought about it. You start not to miss the things you don't have. But once I'd worked my way through the physical challenges and started to come out the other side, I thought that finally we were back on track.

To an extent, we were; however, just as we were starting to re-find our rhythm as a couple, we realised that every other thing that life throws at you as parents gets in the bloody way too. Put together, the utter fatigue, the stress of new and then not-so-new parenthood and trying to work and at the same time respond to the pressures, nice though they are, of our social lives and wider families don't leave much time for reconnecting as a couple. Added to this, while sex was much, much better since I'd started working on my hypertonic pelvic floor and we'd found the joys of lube, it still wasn't always straightforward or spontaneous.

My Story

Like all good things, or maybe all things full stop, it's easy to fall in and out of habits. It takes repetition to make a habit stick, and when you're not doing something, it's even easier to let it slide. Once I'd figured out the root causes of my vaginal pain for penetrative sex, and was on the path to fixing them, I thought that that was it – problem solved!

To an extent it was. The pain was lessening each time we had sex, I felt better in mind and body and we'd figured out which tools we needed to use to make sex more comfortable and pleasurable for us both. We'd worked hard, so hard, on getting to this stage and yes, we had a lot to be proud of. But at times it still felt like there was something missing.

I now see my postnatal journey in three stages: the crisis management phase at the beginning that lasted for about a year, the tail of recovery after that, which went on for two or three years, and the third stage of navigating the rest of parenthood, our relationship, and life's ups and downs, which we're still in, because, as I like to say, once postnatal, always postnatal. As we exited the first stage, I felt buoyant and hopeful that we'd solved a lot of the problems that we needed to in order to work our way back to a fulfilling sex life again. That was partly true, but there was so much more to work on too. What I didn't realise at the time, or perhaps didn't want to acknowledge, was that our wellbeing is a continuum, an ongoing process, a journey that we need to embrace and enjoy rather than seeing the destination as the end goal. Because what is that end goal really? Doesn't it change and shift, shrink and grow as we do?

Firstly, once I'd put out the various physical fires, or at least found the hose and the tap, I started to recognise the need for mental health support too. I've always considered myself quite self-aware, and I thought I knew what I was dealing with and could straighten out the mess in my head by myself. I meditated, I tried to sleep properly, I acknowledged the existential bruises and identity crises I was experiencing. I talked (alright, and argued) a lot with Bryn. I cried and I raged. And I didn't think that I needed anything more. While I've always, always been an advocate for mental health, openness and talking therapy or medication where needed, for some reason I had a mental block when it came to prescribing the same thing for myself.

It took me a year or more to finally acknowledge that things weren't going the way I wanted them to. Despite helping myself to heal in some areas, it was clear that overall there were still things I needed help dealing with. I found a counsellor and started to work through my most obvious symptoms: the anger I couldn't help but show toward my husband and sometimes my daughter, and the guilt and rage I directed toward myself.

I saw that counsellor for a year and realised a great many things. Like the fact that I'd had depression on and off since I was a teenager, that the toxic environment I'd been brought up in was a cause of many of my issues, that I had trouble letting go of things and that my latest bout of rage and guilt, brought on by sheer shock and the changes of pregnancy, birth and the new-new parent period, was postnatal depression impacted by PTSD from the birth.

I had been, I now saw, literally and metaphorically tensing myself through my postnatal depression and entry into a scary new world in which I had no clue what I was doing. This meant that my mental health was affecting my physical health: my shoulders were hunched, my forehead was ever willing to frown, my pelvic floor and core were super tight.

A lot became clearer to me, and home life began to be calmer. But by the end of a year of seeing my counsellor, we'd reached the end of our journey together. This was a lesson for me, too: I thought that once you found a counsellor or therapist, you had to stick with them, but actually when you see a therapist, it's a relationship like any other. And sometimes you outgrow that relationship. A talking therapy partnership is one built on the premise of change and growth. So it's only natural that at some point, you might need to move on. It's not a failure; in a way, it's a success. I felt I could carry on working through things myself, with Bryn and the tools I'd been given. And for a while this was the case. Things looked up and we carried on carrying on.

I should mention that for most of our new parent journey we'd moved away from the place I'd grown up and the place where we had become a couple and started to make our lives: London. After having our daughter, we'd wanted (you guessed it) more space, but couldn't afford it in London. We moved out to the home counties, but not to the place of our dreams. We chose practically and sensibly, opting to be on a train line for the commute, in a manageable house that didn't overstretch us, in a town surrounded by fields, but not with a view. It could have been perfect, and is the dream for many, but for us we missed the vitality of the city, the creative minds that make it buzz, the new cafes popping up on your doorstep and the people who might make us feel at home. As incomers, we found it hard to make friends with people who'd spent most of their lives in the area, and we felt isolated because of that. Without a friendship circle close by and family still in London or even further away, we were putting even more pressure on our marriage, and the arguments abounded, even around the moments of peace.

Over time, the peace withdrew and the arguments got stronger; we were whisper-fighting about divorce on a regular basis. There were silences and stand-offs, and each of us thought the blame lay with the other. We agreed to give it one last try and found a couples' therapist. The first one wasn't right, so we sought another; I think that's important to mention, because when you're bringing someone as potentially contentious as a therapist into your marriage, it's important that that person is right for you both. Like dating, you might go through more than one before you find your match. But Christine was brilliant. Tough but fair, and with a sense of humour that suited us both. We found our sessions draining, cathartic, angry, sad and hopeful. We both cried – him sometimes, me most of the time – and we devoured the food for thought that those sessions gave us.

But in the midst of this progress, I lost a pregnancy. It was an ectopic pregnancy which was removed by keyhole surgery; it was also asymptomatic, which meant that though there had been some unusual (not heavy) bleeding for a few weeks, which wasn't totally unexpected for me, I'd experienced barely any pain. So when I was suddenly and quickly admitted into hospital, it was a shock and left little time for either of us to process. The pregnancy hadn't been planned, but I had been thrilled when two lines appeared on the pregnancy test (in sharp contrast to my reaction the first time round). Bryn was agnostic, which was a disappointment to me. And the unexpected surgical removal brought things into sharp focus.

After the surgery, I was more upset by the experience than I rationally thought I should or would be. It hadn't been longed for, after all. I'd only known I was pregnant for a couple of days, and the thing was still an embryo, not even a foetus. If all had been well, like the first time around, I probably wouldn't have even realised I was pregnant for another month or more. Partly because it was so nascent, so not-yet-a-being, Bryn treated the experience almost like it wasn't happening. And that made it harder for me to process and, unexpectedly, to grieve.

Needless to say, this was more excellent fodder for our couples' therapy, and without Christine, I don't think we would have made it through. With her help, we also established that being in the (sort-of) countryside wasn't working for us. I'd never been sure of the move, and after four years out of the city, Bryn realised that he felt the same. We decided to move back to London, feeling more secure in ourselves now, and clinging on to our marriage as we went.

I also found another personal therapist to help me on the next phase of my journey – one who would work with me to embed self-compassion and nurture my soothing system rather than the drive or fight/flight system that I too often defaulted to (and sometimes still do). For many women, especially mothers, in our pressured society, it's all too easy to forget to soothe ourselves. That's part of the reason why self-care has become such a big watchword. And annoying though it might be to hear people shouting about it all the time (yes, I know I'm one of them), it's actually probably the thing we most need to hear and act upon.

For me, despite all of this improvement, my rage was reaching its peak. And when you're wired to flare up, get ragey, run or *do* at any moment, it's quite hard to find the time to relax into intimacy. It's difficult to connect with yourself, let alone your other half. So as I started to work on my soothing system (and I'm telling you, it's an ongoing journey!), what did that mean for our sex life?

You think, don't you, that having arguments means less sex. That can be true. But what can also be true is that you're living in the same rut you always were and you need the desperate fights and near break-up of the relationship to help you realise that you do like, love and want each other. Or that the discord brings much-needed colour to the boredom and discontent of your everyday life. Or that fighting is somehow separate to, or put on pause to make way for, our sexual interactions. In any case, our sex life wasn't markedly different from how it used to be, but it wasn't anything to write home about. It happened, it didn't feel especially fulfilling, but it wasn't at the top of our priority list to fix it.

The fireworks weren't particularly setting either of our worlds alight. But it's hard, isn't it, to bring that up without offending the other person. To say, "Hey there, you know you used to rock my world and we couldn't keep our hands off each other? Well, you don't anymore." It doesn't matter that you suspect the same is true for them; at the very least you'll probably feel awkward for bringing it up first. And things don't feel catastrophic, so you don't. But you also don't have time for date nights; sometimes it feels like you're running just to keep still.

When to-do lists form the backbone of your daily existence, where does your identity go? Often your identity is subsumed in the detritus of family life, rather than being the spark and the joy of YOU. You don't get turned on, nor do you feel you can turn someone else on. You don't socialise as much (this was especially true in the tough years of the pandemic), so you don't see your other half in a setting with others. When we see our partners with their friends, in a social context, impressing and being impressed, they light up. They're a different person: they're the person you were attracted to when you first met. So when you don't see this for a long time, it's easy to forget why you fancied them in the first place and, conversely, why you might be fanciable yourself.

When you're a mother, your identity is wrapped up in that role. Or it certainly is at the beginning, because it's the defining new factor about you. It's somehow the most powerful label that society puts on us, even though it's not necessarily what we want, or even fair. The thing is that we're mothers first because the reminders of motherhood are all around us. The baby or the kids, the mess, the constant demands on our time, the ever-present echoes of them. Our muffled little internal voices aren't making those demands on behalf of ourselves, and we're not making ourselves heard. Sometimes we can't even hear ourselves, so that time and space disappears. The noise of motherhood is just too loud.

So, What Have We Got Here?

I know you know about all of these, but somehow when you list them and break them down, they become easier to understand, to manage and – dare I say it? – to conquer. Hell, yes.

Lack of Time

I'm talking about time in general (if I don't look at the laundry pile, will it disappear?) and time together. It's really hard as a parent when there are all these new responsibilities on our plate to make time for all the stuff we did before. I'm not saying that this will ever be 100 per cent possible – something has to give, after all – but there's a balance between living like you never had a baby and being subsumed by the diaper mountain.

Be gentle with yourself – at the beginning of your time as new parents, there's a hell of a lot to learn. And wouldn't you know it, all those new things you're doing are a bit bloody tricky when you're doing them for the first time. From getting a baby into a sleepsuit without alerting the whole street, to coaxing a baby to latch without tears on both sides, from keeping on top of all the sick-ups to the actual eons it takes just to leave the house – once you've factored all of these in, there's not a lot of time left over for anything else. And besides, you're exhausted too.

And just when you think you have it nailed, those goddamned babies or kids change again. It's hard to keep up with the new chores that seem to appear at every stage. A baby can literally do nothing for itself, but when your kids are older, free time doesn't necessarily appear in your diary. When they can move, there's more manoeuvring, childcare and after-school clubs to organise, pick-ups and drop-offs to navigate, and more homework, playdates, tantrums and growing intellect to absorb into your schedule.

When your to-do list is hella long, it's no surprise that your sex life might get shoved to the bottom of it. Or even booted off the list entirely. It's normal – I can pretty much guarantee that not everyone else is at it like rabbits. But it's also an area that you can work on if one or both of you are feeling the need for more intimacy. Thankfully, you'll never be quite as clueless as you were the first time you brought a new baby home. You'll get quicker at those chores, and once you've established a routine (excuse me while I laugh to myself), you can make decisions as to what can wait to make room for some sexy time instead. If you have an actual timetable or to-do list (I know you're out there, you super-organisers) why not write it in? Top tip: use code if it's one you keep on the fridge and your in-laws like to peruse it. Otherwise, a little nudge, a text or email from time to time to remind each other that you're not just slaves to your children, can work wonders.

Get Your Mojo Back 101

Dr Emma Svanberg – perinatal clinical psychologist @mumologist

"It's hard to quantify how much, but there are so many influences around us which will impact how we approach sex after birth – not just what we have seen from our parents and how love and intimacy was demonstrated in our family of origin, but also the narratives we have around motherhood and what is 'acceptable' for mothers.

The mental load of motherhood can enormously shrink the space left for desire. Not just because of the practicalities (research has shown that women often feel their role becomes desexualised in long-term relationships or marriage)," plus superscript,[1] but also because there is a great physical load associated with parenting – we don't talk a lot about how physical it can be, and often we might need our bodies not to be touched in order to restore ourselves. I'm sure we can all relate to feeling 'touched out'. It's important to note that hormones play a part as well, as with the drop in oestrogen after birth, so it's not just a mental issue. It's important to bear in mind that there are secondary influences too, because if there is household inequality this can quickly lead to resentment, and of course this can create another barrier to intimacy."

Lack of Connection

When you do eventually find the time and manage to put a date night in the diary, what happens? It can end up being a fizzling disappointment. We look forward to these opportunities so much that expectation can sometimes overwhelm reality. Never mind the problems of getting there in the first place.

If you're breastfeeding, trying to engineer enough time to make it to a restaurant or bar or other date location, have the date and be back in time for the next feed is already exhausting. And then they won't go down when the plan says they should, so you have to shave another 30 minutes off the schedule. Don't burn yourself on the soup! If you're one of those lucky couples who takes the baby with them in the first few hazy months and they sleep under the table, well done! To the rest of you, my commiserations – mine wasn't one of those either. Sleeper or not, they'll soon grow out of this phase, and then you'll have to worry about childcare. You might be able to ask a parent or a relative, but if not, you'll have to: 1) secure a babysitter (good ones are like gold dust) and 2) pay them half your monthly salary for a few hours of questionable peace.

Money is another difficulty. Throwing a baby into the mix can be an expensive business, so finding any spare cash for a date night can be a challenge. Sure, there are cheap and free options, but not always when the baby is able to be handed over, or when you are not working.

Then you can throw the emotional wrench on top of the pile. You've just spent the best part of ten months carrying the baby *inside* you. When it's born, it's usually glued *to* you for much of the day and night. Putting the baby down to go to the bathroom is hard enough, let alone making it out of the house without them. When you get out, that giddy feeling of freedom is a rush on its own. But then you get to the date and you can't stop looking at pictures of your baby on your cellphone/mobile, don't stop talking about that cute/worrying thing they did today, and just *have* to video call the babysitter so you can see they're safely sleeping. Ahem, we did mention that this time was supposed to be for you and your partner, right?

Lack of Forethought and Foreplay

So you've managed to have a date, or some time for yourselves. You decide, against all the odds, to make a break for the bedroom. Yippee! But somehow your mind keeps jumping back to the washing up you haven't done or the laundry that needs taking downstairs, or your ears prick up at the rustle of a snuffling baby in the cot next door. We hold so much in our minds as parents, and we're so alert to our kids as mums, that the amount of cortisol and adrenaline (the primary stress hormones) in our systems can be high and the lack of sleep doesn't help to dissipate these. As you might imagine, cortisol and adrenaline are not quite conducive to a long, relaxed session of love-making. Who knew?

We're also so distracted, and those to-do lists are so long, that it takes a lot to draw back the mind from all those other things. As women, we tend to need our brains to commit to the idea of sex first before our bodies respond, so this can be a problem when we're distracted. Men, on the other hand, tend to experience the opposite. Their bodies react first, and so they're ready for sex more immediately.

What do I mean? Well, desire is the emotional readiness to have sex, whereas arousal refers to the physiological changes that happen to prepare us for sex. Esther Perel believes that women usually need to experience desire before their bodies follow with arousal. This is particularly true in motherhood: "The mother thinks about others the whole time. The mother is not busy focusing on herself. In order to be turned on you have to be focused on yourself in the most basic way."[2] So for females (or those inhabiting the more feminine energy in a relationship), the mind needs to be in the right space in order to kick-start fulfilling sex. This is a problem when everything that's in our heads (domesticity, to-do lists, work, family issues and endless other things) gets in the way of letting our brains relax and stops us giving ourselves over to sex.

When this is the case, it means that for many women, much more time needs to be spent on: 1) building the anticipation, initiating the intimacy, seeding the thoughts and hints of pleasure to come that we need to be able to feel the flicker of desire in the first place; and 2) once the idea of sex becomes established, the amount of so-called foreplay we indulge in to get into the mood. This can be difficult – those damned babies don't sleep for long, after all – and sometimes when we're in a rush, it's hard not to jump straight to the main event.

By "main event", most of us will automatically think of penis in vagina or other penetrative sex. But let's take a moment to ask why foreplay can't be the main event. Why is it dismissively called "foreplay" anyway? Why do language and society put so much emphasis on the penetrative aspect of sex? It's the result of thousands of years of male perspective and draws on some of the points I made in Chapter 1 – namely that animalistically this is the act that allows fertilisation and babies to be made. Now that we are less focused on reproduction, we're able to shift the lens away from men to women, and find pleasure in other ways. And that might mean more foreplay, less penetration; it might mean spending more time on foreplay; it might mean only foreplay. There are no rules regarding what sex is. You can climax or not, you can orgasm without orifices, it can be calm or rough, adventurous or plain vanilla. If you're both getting pleasure out of it, that's enough.

If you're falling short on the desire front, then arousal is often tricky too. Blood might not be flowing to your vagina to give you that tingly feeling, lubrication might not be forthcoming (even more of an issue if your natural lubrication is lacking anyway due to breastfeeding hormones), your clitoris might not be swelling. Add to this the changes in physicality that we've covered in previous chapters, such as scarring, pelvic floor tightness or weakness, lack of sensation and pain, which can make it even harder for desire to break through and arousal to happen. And finally, throw on top even seemingly innocuous parts of us like breasts, which can be over-sensitive from feeding and primed for unexpected milk-jets at the most inopportune times, and aches and pains from all the carrying . . . it's no wonder that we need a little extra time to get in the mood.

The important thing to remember is that all of this is totally fine. Not being able, or wanting, to jump into bed at the drop of a hat and enjoy it is okay. If you're postnatal, your body and mind have been through a lot and are still adjusting. If you're a parent, this shit is hard! This is a different life stage to your Spring Break years, and making allowances for that is more than fine; it's how it should be – it's how we show compassion and, dare I say it, love toward our bodies and ourselves. And you know what? The good thing is that if you work on giving yourself time and grace here, the likelihood is that the sex will improve. Which means you'll probably feel more comfortable and more positive about yourself and your relationship. So you have more sex . . . and it improves again. That's definitely a virtuous circle I can get on board with.

Lack of Sleep

If I've mentioned it once, I've mentioned it a thousand times. The sleep deprivation as a new parent, and even as a not-so-new parent, is real. And right now, I can only wish it were sleep deprivation like I experienced in my twenties. At least I had a good story to go with it then.

The tiredness you experience with newborns is like nothing you've ever known before, and for most of us it's a real smack in the face. It's no surprise that it isn't quite conducive to a rampant night in the sack. When the kids get older, hopefully there's a touch more sleep, but 1) that isn't always the case, and 2) you'll still get the occasional bout of illness, nightmare or random unexplained run of uncooperative children to prevent you from blissfully drifting off to dreamland.

When we're tired our energy is sapped, so we literally have no zest for romance, anyway. All you're thinking about is getting through without killing someone. When your energy is sapped your hackles rise more quickly, and the chances are you'll be snappier than a crocodile and anything but a romance queen. When you're tired, your hormones go out of whack (or even more out of whack than they usually are postnatally) as cortisol and adrenaline flood your body to help get you through.

These stress hormones are not conducive to relaxing into your sensuality and having some couple time.

I recognise that in the overwhelming, confusing and often frustrating times of new parenthood, there is no easy solution to this. Especially if your child is a sleep thief. Believe me, with my second baby, I can relate. So these paragraphs are not a blithe tip to "just get some rest!" – I know it doesn't work like that. But perhaps they can serve as reassurance that what you're going through is understandable and that it can and should get better in the end. Sleep improvement is a slow process and needs consistency. So this is also a reminder to be patient with, and kind to, yourself.

Get Your Mojo Back 101

Dr Karen Gurney, clinical psychologist, psychosexologist and author of *Mind the Gap* @the_sex_doctor

"By far the most common challenge in their sex lives that people come to see me for is discrepancies in desire. In fact, one in four people (men and women) in a relationship don't report the same level of interest in sex as their partner,[3] and this reflects what I see in clinic. Although clients often raise one person's desire as the problem (commonly, they'll say this person, often a female partner if it's a straight relationship, is experiencing low desire), it's almost always a desire discrepancy and therefore something that they both need to work on together.

In terms of the time that it takes to seek help, some people come to see me fairly quickly after problems start. That's actually great, because sometimes challenges around sex can become a little bit more entrenched over time if left unchallenged. But for many people, especially new parents, there are other competing priorities, so it can often be a number of years, or sometimes a number of decades, before people seek help. The main thing to know is that progress can always be made.

After having a baby, I would say there are obviously physical challenges for many people around returning to sex. Painful sex, vaginal dryness caused by breastfeeding and scarring all need time to recover. Despite those things, it's usually challenges to people's psychological wellbeing, and to the relationship's wellbeing, that make it harder for people to return to sex: things like tiredness, stress, overwhelm, panic, adjustment to being a new parent, relationship conflicts that can come with new parenthood and feeling completely touched out. Add to these all of those really obvious other competing priorities, like a lack of time! There are also sometimes relational challenges, including concern over what a partner will think about their changing body, worries that a partner will somehow lose attraction or desire for a mother once they've seen her give birth, or worries that the partner, now that they're a mother, will somehow see them in a less sexual way.

The mental load, tiredness and other competing tasks and priorities affect people much more than they think they should. The reason for that is because desire in long-term relationships is often more responsive. That means it needs nurturing rather than being spontaneous. One of the things that new parenthood does is take away time for desire to be nurtured. So you can't just kind of go from one task like folding away babygros to saying, 'How about sex then?' and expect yourself to feel like it. Often there needs to be time to switch off, there needs to be time for emotional connection and responsive desire to build. With other competing pressures, that can be really challenging. It's not impossible, but it can be really challenging, especially in the first six months to a year after having the baby.

We know from research that people are generally less content with their sex lifes after having children than before.[4] It's common and understandable, given what I've mentioned already. It's rarely the new mothers (and by that I mean the person that's given birth) that comment on being unhappy about the level of sex that they're having, in my experience. More often it's their partners, regardless of their partner's gender, who may feel that this is something to worry about, or that needs addressing. It's probably more common for people who've given birth to worry about their sex life several years down the line, perhaps when they've got a bit more headspace to think about the rest of their relationship and not just parenthood. Immediately after birth, it doesn't seem to be something that mothers raise as much as their partner.

There are three steps that are useful to help people rebuild that intimacy, if that's something that they want to focus on.

The first thing is to understand a little bit more about how desire works. Because generally, as a society, we are in the dark about how desire works in long-term relationships. Being a new parent often means that you're already experiencing the impact of a long-term relationship on your sex life, even before the baby comes along. So understanding that as a couple is the first step.

The second step is to understand from each other what sex brings for you, psychologically. So when you get to sex, what motivates you to do it, how does it make you feel about yourself and the relationship? By knowing that about each other, what you're doing is understanding what happens to the other, and what the threats are to the relationship when one of you feels unconnected sexually. That doesn't necessarily mean that you need to fix that, because it might not be right for you: you might not be able to return to being sexual together at all in any way. But it might mean that you understand a little bit more about your partner. If one of you says, 'it's been a long time since we've had sex, and I'm missing it', that might sound quite irritating. But what they really might be communicating is, 'I feel disconnected from you, I want to know that you still love and desire me.'

It can also make it easier to think about being sexual again when we understand people's motivations and what it is that a partner is missing.

So, the third step, if we're not currently having sex for whatever reason, perhaps because of a new baby or because we're recovering from birth injury, it might be that we can find other ways to make our partner feel connected or desired. For example, setting aside five or ten minutes a week to really connect as a couple, remembering to let them know that you still find them attractive, that you still love them when there are lots of other competing demands."

What Next?

God, it's tough, isn't it? When you are so busy, and so tired, and you just want a nice, easy solution. I know you don't want more tips and advice that takes time to implement. But sometimes the hard way is the best way. Sometimes the habits that we form once we've got over the inertia are the life-changing ones. That's right, life-changing. You heard it here first. So:

• **Put a date night in the diary:** Sure, sure, it's likely to get moved, like, a bajillion times before it happens, but it's in there and it's something to aim for. Experiment with different timings and days. Put in several at once (batch-dating works for us) or one at a time. See what fits into your life. If you batch-date, you can also organise the babysitting at the same time, so you're good to go without the fuss closer to the time. Top tip: the more you do it, the easier it gets, and the more you tend to like one another.

- **Talk:** Yup, I said it. Again. Because I'm telling you, it really does work. If it's not working, it might be because there are some issues you're not raising or maybe it's the end of the road for you, but that's a whole other book right there. I know it's awkward, even if you know and love each other well, or well enough to have kids, but the more you do it, the better you get at it. Introducing sex or intimacy as a topic can be tricky, but 1) it doesn't have to be a formal sit-down: you can lead into it gently; and 2) if you can't talk about sex, how are you going to get the sex you really want and need?
- **Get therapy:** Talking not working or you need a mediator? A counsellor or therapist can be the ideal Switzerland in the bloody battles of your relationship. Not only do they provide a neutral third party who has nothing to gain by taking sides, but they are able to look at your relationship dispassionately and give you a sense of perspective. They're not in the trenches like you are and they're certainly not tied up emotionally in the outcome, so they're able to see clearly and help you find the way to the answers for yourselves. It might not sound like much, but with a good therapist asking the right questions, and a little less hatred and irritation in the room, you might just discover that you actually like one another again – and that's certainly a good first step to wanting to have sex with each other again too.
- **Share the bloody load:** Lord knows we're busy as parents. But, dare I say it, mums are usually busier. Can you parcel out some of the responsibilities so that you're not dealing with them on your own? The less you have on your plate, the more your mind will be able to focus on that little bit of you time you're craving (whether you know it or not). The more time you have for you, the more love you'll have for yourself, the more

confidence you'll build and the more sensual you'll feel. Plus you'll have space in your head for erotic thoughts rather than the grocery list, and that's got to be good for your sex life.

- **Socialise, shock horror, with others:** I know, I know, I've only just told you to go on a date night. Well, when you've managed that one, or maybe even before, take the time to go on an outing with your friends too. A gathering at someone's house, a barbecue or walk, a wedding or party – these are all great places to sneakily observe and admire your partner from a distance, and often that's just the kickstart to your libido that you need. See how he's making them laugh? See how people around you light up when you approach? That's why you fell for each other, and that attraction is still there; it's just a little more buried than you'd like. Take the opportunity to showcase yourselves like you haven't in oh-so-long. This really is a case of distance making the heart grow fonder. You might even find that socialising with others takes the pressure off dates with just the two of you as well, and it should be fun, too, which we all need a little more of as parents.

- **Take yourself out of yourself:** Who are you? What do you stand for? What are you to people now? Those are big questions, and not necessarily ones you can solve with a snap of the fingers. But putting all those questions on pause for just one second can still help. When you have a moment, or during that much-needed self-care or alone time, try to revisit the person you always wanted to be or thought you were going to be. I'm not saying that you need to be that person, but it's good to get a bit of perspective and realise that where you are now doesn't have to be a fixed character. Remember that the sensual and sexual you is buried in there somewhere. Read erotica. Masturbate. Dress up more (even just changing out of that baby-sick-stained top is helpful) and put a little make-up on (a swipe of lippy or mascara can do wonders) if that's your thing. Try to reconnect with who you were, and who you ARE, without all that kid crap and baby paraphernalia around you.

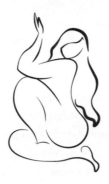

THE FATHERLOAD

*Exploring the experience
of dads and partners.*

Although this book is driven by my own experience and my
mission is to make sure your journey as a new mum and a woman
is more comfortable, empowered and positive (hooray for us!), for
many of us there's another person in the mix too. Our (hopefully)
supportive other halves are there for us throughout the journey,
and they're in this equation too. I've talked about couple dynamics,
teamwork, communication and more throughout the book,
but in this chapter I want to focus on the partner's perspective,
because we can sometimes become too focused on our own point
of view. Let's be fair, we don't often get too much dedicated focus
as mums, and I'm totally for looking after ourselves (let me hear
it for self-care!), I just want us to avoid complete tunnel vision. A
lot of this chapter also applies to same-sex partners and partners
who are not the father of your baby.

　While women are the ones who experience childbirth,
in whatever form, and its associated identity shift, dads and
partners also have to adjust with us. It can be a HUGE change
for us, but it can also be extremely significant for our other
halves. In some cases the shift to parenthood leads to mood

disorders like postpartum depression or postpartum anxiety, but partners (men in particular) can be even less likely than we are to speak openly about the impact that new parenthood has on their identity and mental health. For men especially, a society which still broadly values strong and silent masculinity doesn't exactly leave much headroom for a deep and meaningful conversation. For same-sex partners, the focus is still on the one who has given birth. Yes, I know it's changing, but there are still some traditional hang-ups which are hard to get rid of.

And, while sex is fabulous solo, it's also a team activity, one which can often be the glue at the heart of your relationship. Becoming parents affects both of you and has a knock-on effect on your sex life: this chapter explores how partners experience the shift to parenthood. It dives into how it might look and feel from their perspective in terms of the mental and physical shift itself, how it impacts their approach to sex and how it can feel for them when witnessing our sometimes difficult journey.

I'm going to talk about how our other halves can feel when we're going through all this shit, because it can be pretty tricky on the other side of the convo too. Perhaps they feel helpless in the face of a whole new whirlwind of emotions, powerless and confused in the face of symptoms that they never realised would be a problem. Maybe they're even losing their mojo due to the loss of their own mental wellbeing.

Yes, postnatal depression in dads is a thing: around eight to ten per cent of men (in homosexual and heterosexual couples) get it.[1] And get this: if you as the mother are going through mental health difficulties, your other half is up to 50 per cent more likely to experience postnatal depression themselves.[2] Woah. That's not insignificant, and while as a society we're now doing much better at addressing mothers' mental health, we have a way to go in fostering the same openness toward fathers' mental health. There are currently fewer studies for same-sex couples, but lesbian partners seem to be less at risk of depression and anxiety than their carrying partners.[3] But for most of us, if you add together the levels of mental health in both partners, the resulting combined libido probably isn't going to be sky high!

While reduced sex may be driven on the new mum's side by (a totally understandable) lack of desire due to, for example, breastfeeding or vaginal pain, recent studies have confirmed that it's also due to your partner experiencing that same stress, fatigue and lack of time.[4] To me, this makes a whole lot of sense, as dads and partners are taking on much more of an equal role as parents – and thank goodness for that.

The changes in men are not just physical and mental, but also physiological. Many new fathers see a fairly significant drop in testosterone that can cause erectile dysfunction. We're used to thinking of the mother's physiology and hormone levels changing, but along with a drop in testosterone, a study based in the Philippines found the presence of prolactin (yes, *that* prolactin) in fathers up until the baby was around one year old.[5] Aren't bodies amazing?

I think it's also safe to assume that our partners' feelings of failure or overwhelm if there's a drop in libido, difficulties with arousal or lack of sexy time can be as strong as those that we're feeling ourselves. I'm mentioning all of this because it contributes to our overall sexual wellbeing as a couple, and because I think it reduces the onus on us as mothers to get ourselves fixed – it's a group effort. Teamwork makes the dream work, after all, so getting your partner on board with this journey, in both increasing your understanding of each other's perspective and taking practical steps to help you both heal, will mean you'll reach your destination much more quickly.

Let's Hear from my Husband

My husband, Bryn, has been a rock for me throughout our relationship. That rock hasn't been without its hidden edges and unexpected curves (because what relationship is perfect?), but the foundation of our relationship and the commitment that we made a long while ago is strong. Which is handy, because in the words of those trusty swedish pop sages, ABBA, "Love isn't easy, but it sure is hard enough." We've managed, after years of self-development and counselling, both together and apart, to reach a place where we can successfully communicate with each other – but it hasn't always been straightforward.

I wasn't brought up to be an emotional talker. We didn't say sorry in my house; we shouted and then acted like nothing had happened. And that means when Bryn and I bicker (okay, fight), I find it really hard to apologise and admit when I'm in the wrong. I would much rather ignore it than talk about it. In the beginning, communication on that level was stilted. It still wasn't easy when we had our first daughter, and it certainly became even more challenging when we experienced all the issues that led to this book. So I want you to hear from Bryn, because it was a journey for him too; this has helped me see that in some ways, my experiences were actually joint experiences and they impacted us both.

It's a real-life view, and I think it's important for us all to get an understanding of the other side of the coin, particularly because it helps to highlight how teamwork and talking helped us navigate our (let's be honest here) mess.

Bryn's Story

Did I have any understanding of postnatal sex prior to Clio giving birth the first time? No. I think I was so focused on all the other stuff like the birth, being a dad and having a small child. We'd covered episiotomy in the antenatal classes, so I had some concept that there'd be some physical healing needed, but I don't remember having thought about the emotional healing and the relationship between physical and emotional rehabilitation at all. I was also under the impression that if you had a "normal" birth, then the vagina would be fine afterwards; I had no concept of stretched muscles or bruising, and thought a tear or a cut, for example, would be traumatic and need more looking after. I guess I thought "the body is meant to do this", and therefore healing should be easy.

Postnatal sex doesn't make it to the top of the list of conversations to have pre birth, does it? In among all of the talk about how you're going to keep the baby alive, sex felt like more of a grey area. I knew it would be different, but I thought we'd get to it when we got to it. You obviously do know of people who have two kids 12 months apart . . . so you know that sex is possible! But they're probably the ones you hear about – you don't hear about the stories like ours where the couple didn't have sex for a year because it was too painful, either mentally or physically.

Postnatal care definitely falls between the gaps in terms of maternity care. If you're dying, the NHS is great: it's the bits around the edges that are dropped. And the number one priority with antenatal stuff is to get you through the birth and keep the baby alive. So there often isn't any room for formal training or teaching on anything postnatal – it sits in that "nice to have" category that there's never a budget for. With postnatal sex in particular, it's even trickier. There's something uniting in the stuff about the baby; all couples want to keep the baby alive and do the right thing, whereas sex lives are different and personal. I can imagine some people thinking, "It's just too awkward and not what I bargained for." What's annoying, though, is that all of this "nice to have" stuff is actually preventative – a lot of the time the healthcare system would save a hell of a lot of money by informing people beforehand and helping them to take care of themselves.

I was surprised too that Clio wasn't given any information about scarring or pelvic floor rehabilitation after the birth; it was never suggested that she should see a women's health physio. She didn't get any advice about massaging her scars either, which I find particularly weird: it's such a zero cost.

Often formal care ends, and then your community network and family takes over. But with sex, it's not a topic that people are really talking about – a bit like miscarriage. It should be passed down through stories and families and culture and life, as well as through medical professionals: received wisdom through the generations. But it's not, because it's seen as taboo. I wonder if there could be more openness in society around postnatal sex like there is around miscarriage these days. Both medical help and awareness can be powerful, because you need awareness to know you need help, and then you need the medical provision to exist to get it sorted.

In terms of my own conversations with friends, I've touched on it with my closest friends, in that we probably mentioned something about how long it was before we had sex again, and whether that was easy or difficult, or something like that. So, without details. Which means it's a fine line between walking the walk of passing down received wisdom and respecting the reality of people's willingness or unwillingness to talk. As my friends are also conscious of their partners' privacy, it's a tricky cycle to break.

My default assumption is that bad stuff won't happen to me, so I wasn't overly worried about what sex after the birth would be like for us. When it did happen and I saw the reality of the bleeding afterwards, the pads and the pain and Clio not being able to get up and move around . . . I'm not sure I was prepared for the extent of that: they say you will be sore, but it's one thing to hear it and another thing to experience it.

My nervousness was heightened by the fact that Clio's body had been through something while mine hadn't.

So in terms of initiating sex, it really just felt in no way in my court, and certainly inappropriate to be pushing for it! On the other hand, I think Clio wanted to prove that she could have sex, like everything was back to normal, but the first time was distressing. I knew she was going to be sensitive, physically and emotionally. And I think we'd had times as well, even before that, when sex had not gone well, which had upset her. We can laugh about it now, but perhaps we should have been a bit more circumspect at the time, especially as I think the whole experience was caught up with Clio's depression as well. I tried my best to be supportive, but she just didn't want to be told that it would be alright, because it wasn't. Our communication wasn't good at that point either. There were lots more layers to it than either of us realised at the time.

What's upsetting is that it usually gets left as the woman's problem. It's easy for me to say "Don't worry, it'll be alright", because I'm not left thinking "What's wrong with me? Is it this or this? Should I do this or this now?" Men can feel like they're being quite patronising for trying to solve that problem while not really knowing what the problem is.

I think I was surprised by how long it took to find an answer. I was surprised by how long it took and how hard it was for Clio to find it, and then how simple the answer was in the end. There was a long healing process even after finding the answer, though: the massage and desensitisation that Clio had to do as well as working on the traumatic associations between sex and childbirth took some time. It's all very well for me to sit here saying, "Oh, it was really simple in the end", but that's the benefit of hindsight!

In terms of the impact on me emotionally, I don't think I had a particularly strong sexual identity at that point in my life; I probably still don't. Which was helpful in a way, because I didn't feel a threat to my identity or to my self-worth. What it did do was contribute to a picture of things being wrong between us, which obviously affected me a lot, because I ended up with insomnia and anxiety. These symptoms were triggered by a change in job a year or so later, but all the conditions were there right from the start of the postnatal period.

Funnily enough, I don't remember either our relationship or intimacy and sex being really distressing until we moved out of London. We were just about getting some sleep at that point, and we were settled in a house and perhaps we both just started to think it would be nice to start having sex again, but it was still difficult. I always felt sex was more about satisfying my partner than about me, so not being able to be intimate in the same way didn't distress me in the same way it distressed Clio, but it was upsetting.

It definitely contributed to the difficulties in our relationship. Our problems with sex played into a narrative that things in our marriage were broken. It reinforced that things weren't working. And the lack of communication was really hard. It seemed to be yet another thing that we couldn't work out how to discuss. I also felt criticised for lots of things in that period, and my response to that was that this was yet another thing I wasn't getting right. In a way, the postnatal sex issue was a microcosm of the broader relationship: sex was another wedge in the marriage. Every time we tried to do something and failed, be it agree on a holiday, put on a birthday party or have sex, we argued. It didn't help that Clio likes to be in control and doesn't like to fail. I was also totally uncomfortable with failure. So, when something went wrong, it seemed like a much bigger deal. And it did feel like failure, because Clio was so vocal about it being a failure. I'm not sure I would have felt so bad about things if I were left to my own devices. But it did mean that we both felt responsible, so perhaps in a way it led to us trying to find a solution.

Eventually I reached a point in our marriage where I thought that it was either going to get better or it was going to end, which would also have been better than the way things were! I reached rock bottom before Clio did, I think, and certainly before we went to couples' therapy. I lost my fear of divorce, and once I lost my fear of it, it kind of didn't matter anymore. I lost my fear of confrontation and learned to stand up for myself at some point quite a long time before therapy; I found that really liberating. But obviously therapy was the big turning point and determined which of those two paths we took.

It wasn't immediately obvious what the outcome would be, though. I think I was still protecting myself – Clio was much more hopeful about what couples' therapy would give us, but I was definitely 50:50 at the beginning.

We were both seeing therapists before we started couples' counselling, so I can't really think why we hadn't done it before. I remember thinking we both had our own issues that we needed to work on, and believing there was sense in doing it separately – like we just individually needed to be happy and then we would both be happy. It's hard to be happy as a couple if one of you isn't. I didn't feel like there was stigma around couples' therapy – and definitely not with individual therapy, because it's so close to self-improvement, which I love! But I think there are definitely different ways of using therapy these days. Whereas traditionally you might see it as more of a last chance saloon, now some of it is more preventative, like a relationship MOT, and that can be really beneficial too.

Therapy gave us a different perspective and way of communicating. We're definitely not perfect now, but it is better. Not in the way that people might think. It's not as if as soon as there's an issue we sit down and one of us calmly raises it with the other. It's more that we understand each other's languages now. We both understand we're probably going to fight in certain circumstances. I understand that if Clio is sniping at me, it's unlikely to be wholly because of me (but probably partly because of me) and also that something else might be going on. And we both understand that it's important to tell the other if we're feeling depressed or anxious much earlier than we would have done before.

I would emphasise that it's about understanding as much as communication. It's about reading what is being said as much as what is being meant. So the communication might be sniping, but I really know that what is meant is, "I'm not in a great place." That makes a world of difference and really helps us to feel better connected, which obviously helps us to like each other, and ultimately want to be intimate.

Going through the whole fatherhood experience, I think just knowing that birth isn't always a full mother nature experience is really important for your relationship afterwards. Society gives us default assumptions of the "natural" birth process – that the body is meant to do this, and therefore if it is just given time, it will heal, and everything will just happen. But actually there is stuff you can actively be doing to support and rehabilitate which can make everything a whole lot better for you both.

It's a nice soundbite to say the onus shouldn't always be on the woman [in birth and the postnatal period], but it's hard for the onus to be on the man. The biggest thing I've learned is that it's not enough to just be supportive; you have to be knowledgeable too. I put a higher priority on being informed at the birth of our second daughter. I think of myself as a supportive person, but it's a bit useless without knowledge. It's all very well being there, but asking "What do you want me to do?" is not helpful and probably quite irritating for your partner.

I'm really proud of opening up the conversation about sexuality in motherhood and as parents, because on a basic level, talking about sex is awkward, embarrassing. It's always easier to talk about something else or even go and do the washing up. But I also think that men in general (maybe I'm atypical) develop quite narrow sexual identities. I imagine a woman's sexual identity to be quite round, like a ball, and a man's as linear. It has less depth or richness to it in terms of what you enjoy, or where you enjoy it, or what it feels like. It can be quite black and white, and come down to whether you are pleasing your partner or not. So I think for men, conversation about sex is going to be awkward, but that's because it happens from a place of asymmetry, where you have women with quite developed sexual identities and men with two-dimensional sexual identities; but I think it's important for us all to work on that so we can be fulfilled and happy.

Teamwork Makes the Dream Work

Or, as I like to say, there's no point in cutting out your partner (if you have one) on this postnatal sex journey. They might not have experienced the birth, mental and physical changes that you have, but they're there (hopefully) to make things easier for you. Sharing is caring, and getting your other half on board with where you are, as well as understanding what they are experiencing, is a key ingredient in this recipe of lurve. You know the mantra "There is no 'I' in team", right?

However, in the case of postnatal sex and enjoying intimacy long into a marriage or relationship as parents, it's also vital that we sort out the "I" alongside sorting out our shit as a team. Think about it: so much of what we're going through in the early parenthood period, both physically and mentally, is personal; and yet so many of our intimate experiences are with someone else. Doesn't quite translate, does it? And that's because really, you both need to understand what each of you is going through, be comfortable with it and forgiving of yourselves and be able to rehab and heal properly so that you can bring your best selves to the bedroom party. Put it this way: spending time on ourselves first is like making sure we get the best ingredients for our recipe, and then prepping them well (that's your rehab and recovery), so that our casserole will taste all the better for it at the end. I think I'm making myself hungry.

It's also worth pointing out that you can, and will, have amazing, pleasurable intimacy again (whether solo or together), and your partner can be part of the formula to help you get there. The weight is not all on your shoulders. Thank fuck for that. Here are some things to think about.

Communication

It can make some of us (ahem, mentioning no names) feel uncomfortable, but communication really is the key to getting what you both need out of your relationship. As a concept, it's not the sexiest answer you're looking for, I know, but some of these examples of how to implement it might be.

- **Turn it into a game:** Communication isn't quite the sort of game you ever thought you'd be playing as a teenager, but when the state of your marriage is the prize, isn't it worth giving it a go? If you feel awkward about it, there are several card games which promote good conversation, some of them designed specifically for couples, which are an excellent prompt for a simple chat or a deep and meaningful conversation. I've listed a few of them at the end of the book under this chapter's resources, but there are plenty out there these days – have a search and see what sort of style might suit you best. In our experience, you just need a few cards to get the ball rolling, and more often than not it leads to an actual topic you came up with yourself. Once you've played it a few times, you'll be old hands at this conversation lark, so why not make a few prompt cards of your own? Make a note of the questions that got those jaws moving and save them for future sessions.

- **Eat face to face:** Yeah, I know, mind-blowing concept. But how often do we eat separately, standing up, grabbing something one-handed when we can and wolfing it down as quickly as possible before the baby wakes? When was the last time you sat down to eat or used an actual plate? Who remembers cutlery?! Even into later parenthood, the speed-eating tendencies are hard to kick; I had just about slowed down to pre-kid digestion after my first daughter when my second came along. My first was already seven years old. Anyway, petty interruptions to a relaxing dinner can take the form of waking children (bedtimes aren't always straightforward even past the toddler years), school and work stresses and any and all of life's big and small irritations. And I don't know about you, but there are plenty of times during the week when we eat on the sofa in front of Netflix. All of this adds up to one less opportunity to sit and talk, and know where your partner is at. So if you can, make a point of sitting down together, just the two of you, once a week over dinner (or lunch or breakfast, if those mealtimes are easier to manage with childcare, work or tantrum schedules). If it turns into a habit, so much the better.

- **Go for a walk or drive:** If the good old face-to-face isn't getting you anywhere, or is bringing up more negative vibes than positive, it can be easier to talk when you're not looking at the other person. It feels somehow private but you still have a direct line to their ear, so it takes the pressure off. Sometimes we can feel easily embarrassed by tricky conversations, or even at the thought of them. Though they don't have to be tricky, conversations about our sex lives usually do fall into this category. Even if we know we shouldn't be embarrassed (you're not alone in experiencing it, by the way, but you should be proud that you recognise the need to talk), society treats sex as a subject to be laughed about, or to shame us for or to brush under the carpet entirely. So start gently with a walk. Or have a chat while you're going on a drive. Somehow when you're doing something else, the focus is softened and you're not under quite such a bright spotlight.

- **Ask your friends:** Look, I'm not saying that they're going to share all the intimate details of their relationship or bedroom antics with you, but you'd be surprised, when you ask them outright and tell them what's going on with you, just how many of your friends are going through similar things and can relate. It might not provide you with any answers, and nor should you expect it to – our relationships are all unique – but it will serve as a great reminder that we're not alone. If you *both* do this, you'll also probably get perspectives from both partners in a relationship, so neither of you will feel put upon or maligned. I cannot emphasise enough how important normalising the ups and down of our relationships is: life doesn't end at "I do". Deciding to be together, getting married, having a baby, none of that guarantees a happily ever after. Recognising when there are issues and working on them might.

- **Build a compassion bank:** We're often barely compassionate toward ourselves, particularly as parents, and it's exacerbated in Western societies that value getting on with it, working hard and progressing. We spend so much of our time prioritising the small people, it's hard to make room in our cluttered mental attic for ourselves. We truck on. But when we truck on, not only does it suggest to others that we're fine and don't need looking after, but we also absorb that rhetoric for our own internal narrator. So ask yourself: can you start by being a bit more compassionate toward yourself? I guarantee you that if you can start doing this, others will tend to follow. And when you communicate that this is your goal, you might just find that your other half will come along for the ride too. It works both ways. If you both feel you need to show more kindness toward yourselves and to each other, why don't you both give it a go? You know that saying "walk a thousand miles in someone else's shoes"? It's that, but less twee. Cultivating a compassionate view will help take the pressure off you, whether it's coming from within you or from external sources, especially at a fragile time. I promise you there is magic in learning to convey your needs, not being embarrassed by them *and* in listening to and acting on theirs. That's definitely team work right there.

Get Your Mojo Back 101

Dr Emma Svanberg – perinatal clinical psychologist @mumologist

"Often becoming parents is the first time in our lives that we have experienced such stark role differences due to gender, especially if we are in a heterosexual relationship. Our days can suddenly feel very different, and we are negotiating huge changes in every area of our lives. Mothers can also feel more in need of looking after themselves, and if your relationship has not been based on this previously, it can feel difficult to know how to ask for this or whether it will be received well. We don't tend to talk beforehand about how we are going to manage these transitions, and as a result many couples can feel that they are drifting. There can be an awkwardness to discussing relationships in general if this isn't something that you have done before – needing to assert your needs and expectations and find compromise about how daily life will be. We are also often time-poor as parents, and exhausted, and it can be difficult to articulate these issues.

When it comes to sex in particular, there are so many obstacles that get in the way of open communication. Desire is very often based around mystery, and new parenthood can really blow that apart! So having to figure out how to talk about your sexual relationship in a new way can feel challenging. We – men and women – might also find our libido has been affected by becoming a parent, and worry about the impact rejection has on our partners. All of these things can create increasing barriers that feel harder to get over the longer they go on.

Sometimes the father's [or partner's] role can inhibit his sexuality just as motherhood can for women, perhaps depending on the expectations he has placed on himself about what a good dad and partner is. Issues such as postnatal depression in the father/partner or the mother, or witnessing a traumatic birth, can also impact on sexual desire. However, there are gender differences in how all-encompassing parenthood can be. Women are often encouraged (unconsciously or explicitly) to abandon the parts of themselves which are unrelated to motherhood – a loss of their subjectivity. For men, there is not the same pressure to do this, and as a result it is more likely that they can hold on to the sexual parts of their identity. Society often ignores men's mental health or emotions more broadly and men can absolutely struggle with the identity shift toward fatherhood too. We talk more now about matrescence [a woman's shift into the motherhood phase]. Even though it is still not enough, there is support around and understanding about the transition to motherhood. There is not the same conversation about the transition to fatherhood, and in so many ways this perpetuates the idea that parenting is really only the concern of women."

His and Hers

As Bryn talked about above, it's pretty tough for partners to walk the line when it comes to the whole postnatal sex conversation. Because our partners haven't been through our experience. Yes, they may have seen it, they may have been there with you, probably even held your hand . . . but that doesn't always add up to understanding. In our case, while Bryn was keen to help and could see how much I was struggling, he didn't feel qualified to comment or suggest solutions with anything like authority. And with the mental state I was in, I was in no mood to entertain his tentative ideas about a way forward.

So when we swap places and it comes to our understanding of what our partner is going through, it might be a surprise that the waters can still be muddy. We (usually) love our partners and want to acknowledge their experience, but we might not be in a position to truly appreciate it. And when it comes to how they're feeling about sex and exploring sensuality again, we might not be able to second guess how they're feeling either.

The Word on the Street

Bryan, 70, dad and grandfather

"I wasn't surprised that there would be issues with postnatal sex. I was at the birth of our firstborn and, being interested in seeing the actual delivery, I was quite shocked to see what an episiotomy entailed. And I remember thinking, 'That pair of scissors looks blunt to me.' Then I thought 'This is my wife's most sensitive area being cut' and there was also a tear quite far into the perineum. So I was aware of the damage to her vagina and perineum and I certainly remember worrying about this when we decided to have sex again after the birth.

However, I had little experience of vaginal dryness and had never used a lubricant for sex. Prior to our marriage in the mid-1970s (and with the 20/20 vision of hindsight), I don't think I talked sensitively enough with my male friends about our sexual encounters. There was probably a bit too much light-hearted banter; I don't think men are 'led to believe certain things' [about sex after birth], but when you have watched a vaginal birth at close quarters, it is obvious that there will be some changes and these may be experienced by both partners."

What Next?

Of course, now you've mastered the communication that we talked about just now, you'll probably be laughing all the way to the intimacy bank, but if you still need a little reminder and a helping hand, let's get practical: here's how to improve that understanding of what the other is going through and feeling.

We've talked a lot about our own desires and intimate needs. How do we factor in our partner's desires and needs too? And how do we ensure they fit with our own journey? Before you start worrying that I've lost the plot – "What's changed for them?!" – bear in mind that they have made a great leap forward into parenthood too, and that transition is (as you know) tough. They are probably also impacted, at least on a certain level, by watching how you're making that transition; they care about you and you care about each other. Let's do this together. Because actually, you might find that what I'm about to suggest can help you rediscover your own wants too. Can't say fairer than that.

- **How will I know?** If you're channelling Whitney vibes, the best thing to do is *ask*. It's not rocket science. You can't see into their head and they can't see into yours. You might have become pretty good at reading each other by now, but what if you've read it wrong? Ask how they feel about having sex again. *If* they feel like having sex again. When they might want to give it a go. What sort of sex that might be (it's not all about penetration). What they're worried about. Whether they're turned on by different things now. How you're actually going to make it happen or find the time. Oh, and don't forget you need to feed into the conversation with your thoughts too.

- **Listen:** Before you go leaping in at the deep end when there's a hint that things might not be working, take a second and breathe. No one likes to know that they're falling short of the mark, but this isn't a test; it's not a judgement on you, and any changes and gentle nudges in a different direction do not malign what came before. Are things feeling out of kilter for you too? Here's the place to bring it up. You might find that rather than taking you back a step, listening to each other and re-engineering the formula might leave you much better off in the sexual stakes than you were even before bub came along.

- **Suggest:** You're reading this book. I reckon that means you're pretty in touch with your sensuality, or at least the possibility of rediscovering it and improving your sex life. So once you've listened, make some suggestions. I'm not saying take over the conversation (give and take, remember), but if it seems as if they're struggling to find the right words or they feel embarrassed to be asking, why not throw out a few ideas yourself?

You might find you're the knowledgeable one, or the one who feels more empowered around sensuality. Use that to help bring your partner's needs out too. The good thing is that you can bring your own desires into the picture too, especially now that your, and their, arousal prompts may have changed. This helps frame the conversation, a bit like word association – their immediate response to something that you suggest might give you a starting point and let you know if it's something they might be into or they're 100 per cent not into. By working out what you both really want or don't want, you can both learn to express your desires in a healthy way. You're not going to know how to light their fire, and they're not going to know how to light yours if you don't talk about it.

- **Compromise:** Forget the Art of War: if there's an Art to Marriage, it's compromise. That's true when you're bickering over the washing up or thrashing out childcare schedules, and when it comes to the bedroom. If you've learned nothing else in this book (though I'll be honest, I really hope that's not the case!), then compromise is a pretty good takeaway all by itself. You might want X, they might want Y. That's fine. Try one and then the other. Or if X really doesn't work for one of you, help each other to vocalise why and find another way. A good example of this is any kind of penetrative sex – you might be tentative because of the pain, they might be tentative because they're aware of how much your body's been through and they don't want to bruise it further. You might find your fears are unfounded, or you might realise that non-penetrative sex is actually what floats your boat right now. Figure out where your desires lie and figure out what's best for both of you.

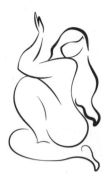

TAKE TWO

Trying for subsequent babies, and sex after trauma and loss.

Trigger Warning: this chapter contains discussion of baby and pregnancy loss, and sexual assault.

Often, when you've finally got the hang of baby number one, your thoughts will turn to having number two; it's not uncommon for families to have two children under two years old these days, which means that many probably start thinking about getting pregnant when their baby is just a year old. Depending on your experience, you might think this is a bit of a surprise really, given how utterly mind-blowing (in both good and bad ways) that first year can be. Think about it: your life is finally coming back together, you're starting to feel like your old self, but sure, why not throw another pregnancy and postnatal period into the mix?!

Sex is really the pinch point in this decision. If you've struggled with any of the physical and mental issues that we've been discussing so far, it might be a touch surprising that you'd feel ready to go through it again. If you are, then fabulous for you. If you're not, then that's totally okay too. With sex potentially causing so many issues after the first birth, it's hard to envisage just how we get pregnant again. You might not want to have sex for a long time if it's been painful or you have birth injuries. You might not feel able to associate pleasure with your vagina after trauma. You might struggle with the transition to motherhood and be going through mental health issues. You might not want to take on even more chaos and overwhelm. You might not (and this is the big one) be able to find the ruddy time.

Add to this the pressure of "trying" again, and the joy that you have managed to cultivate again for intimacy suddenly disappears. Things can be further impacted when we consider sex after a birth layered with baby loss, sex after pregnancy loss, sex after a rainbow baby via a struggle with infertility, sex after assault, sexual aggression or even rape. Sex can be wonderful and empowering, beautiful, intimate and connection-forming. But these experiences can undermine all of those things too.

And yet somehow it happens. Most of us do overcome all these things. So if that's the right decision for us, how do we find the time and pleasure to have sex in the context of all the issues that we've talked about? It's hard enough to marry the idea of sexuality and motherhood the first time around, so how do we throw ourselves into it all over again? This chapter unpacks a little further how these experiences can impact our feelings and approach toward sex in these contexts, and scratches the surface of how we can start to move on or resolve them, finding the beauty and connection in intimacy again.

Deciding to Try Again

As you've probably understood by now, I had some issues to deal with vis-à-vis sex after birth. We've discussed the physical and mental ramifications of going through childbirth and the difficulties of finding the right way to rehabilitate. We've also talked about how difficult it is to find even a sliver of time and the inclination to have sex again in parenthood. In my case, all of the things that we went through as a couple meant that we didn't start having fulfilling sex again until two years after I gave birth. Then we found that sex just wasn't the feature it had been earlier in our relationship. We were doing okay. If we had issues as a couple, it wasn't solely because of the amount of sex we were having! But it was only at three years postpartum that I felt ready to *consider* trying for another baby. Frankly, it had been a hard "no" up until that point. The year after that was about wavering and discussing – for us, having another baby was a big decision. When we did start trying, at four years, it took a little while to get pregnant, and then I suffered an ectopic pregnancy . . . All of which we probably didn't expect would be part of our journey to a family of four. We do have a second daughter now, and in this chapter I'll talk a little more about how we actually got there.

My Story

Getting through my first birth and the resulting fall-out was one of the hardest things I've ever had to do, if not the hardest. I know that for many couples the decision to have another baby (or not to) is an easy one. Many women I know have a fairly concrete idea, if not an actual plan carved in stone, of how many children they want to have and when, of how their family will look when it's complete. There are also a great many of us on the other side of the coin who don't. Perhaps you have a vague idea, but you're not tied to it. Or you have an idea but then real life happens, and suddenly you're not so sure any more.

And by "life", I mean things like the experience of your first birth, an infertility journey, baby or pregnancy loss and sexual assault or rape. These are, of course, incredibly different in their own ways and in the impact that they'll have on you. I don't mean to lump them in together, truly. But what they all have in common is that they throw us off course. They impact our perception of, and joy during, sex. They knock our self-confidence and identity. They make us scared and ashamed. And they also impact how and whether we decide to have another child. If and when we do choose to go for a subsequent baby, they throw us curveballs; they change how we feel about sex, pregnancy and birth and how we approach the journey. And I'm not just talking about the sex that we need to get pregnant again. All of these things can impact our enjoyment of sex altogether. They mess with our minds on the role of our sexuality, how comfortable we are with sensuality in general and the role it has to play in our relationships.

I found it incredibly intrusive and frustrating when people would keep asking, "So when are you going to have another one then?" Or comment jovially, "Well, you don't want to leave it too long do you?" Or even the judgemental, "Ah, you can tell she's an only child, she needs a sibling really, doesn't she?" I wanted to scream at them. I dreamed of shouting back, in the street to complete strangers and also at family gatherings to close relatives who really should know better, "You don't know me! You don't know what I've been through."

I thought, and I still think, that people should recognise that people have their reasons and try to be sensitive to that. Unfortunately, they don't always understand this, particularly if they haven't been through similar things themselves. Without the perspective of experience, people don't realise that their throwaway comments are actually nosy. In my case, they made me feel guilty and ashamed about my decision. Who'd have thought there were so many layers to an innocent conversation filler?

I did feel guilty. I felt the pressure, both internally, because I like to be in control and feel that my life is "on track", and externally, because everyone I knew had (or was on their way to having) two kids. I saw peers and other mothers on social media who had found birth easy, or at least pretended they had, or had sprung back from the hit like a prize fighter, ready to take on more. Whereas I felt bruised, wounded and not at all sure of myself. I was hurt and wanted to protect myself, and I wasn't at all sure whether going back for more in the form of a second pregnancy and child was the right thing to do.

Besides, there was a lot of healing to do. One thing at a time, I thought. I managed to get help and the right rehab for my pelvic floor. Tick. I managed to admit I needed help with my mental health and begin to work through those issues. Tick. We managed to swerve divorce and maintain a marriage. Tick. We managed to keep a child alive, happy and healthy. Tick. Did I really want to go and mess it all up by putting us through it all again by trying to have another baby?

The thing is, when you wait to have a second child, you get past all the shit stuff. The truly sleepless nights, the nappies, the teething pain, the weaning mess, the potty-training, the total and utter energy-sapping reliance on you. And you make it out the other side to a child that can really do quite a lot for themselves. Suddenly (or not so suddenly) you have a little person who is great fun to be around, can read, write and hold a decent conversation, and if you're lucky, they might even occasionally bring you a cup of tea. So, the fact that we would be staring down the barrel of starting completely from scratch, doing it all over again, made the thought of having another baby even more daunting.

So where were we? Well, we'd both always thought we'd have more than one child. We both have siblings, and I guess I liked the idea of our daughter having a buddy. Bryn had still been keen on the idea after

Delphi was born, but as time went on, we both became more comfortable with the idea of sticking with one. We had a lot to think about, and I wasn't ready to be pregnant for such a long time after the first birth that it became more of a vague and small possibility than a firm idea. My associations with birth and the postnatal period were all negative and hard for me to process: I was hurting for a long time. We both were.

But time is a great healer. They say that mothers' memories of birth fade, otherwise we'd never have another. Perhaps there's some truth to that, because although I didn't forget completely, it definitely began to feel more manageable. I'd found a way to rehab and get through it after all, hadn't I? Perhaps it could be done again. For the first two years after birth, I would say "absolutely no way" when people asked if we'd have another. By the end of that two years, I (we) began to feel the positive effects of the rehab and healing work, and hope began to reassert itself. Sex wasn't so painful, and we began to reconnect. I was getting therapy and beginning to own and deal with the issues that made me so angry and depressed. The trauma of the birth began to feel like something I could cope with. Motherhood became less overwhelming.

In that third year, we talked, tentatively, about whether a second child was right for us. We didn't come to any conclusions, but it wasn't something that I baulked at automatically anymore. When, after another year, we did decide to start trying, it took a while to get pregnant, unlike the first time round. And looking back on it now, I realise that actually I was on tenterhooks about it. We weren't going into it carefree and happy, perhaps we weren't even sure it was the right thing to do. Maybe Bryn just didn't have the words to tell me that he thought it was a bad idea. I don't mean to be a cliché, but I think on some level I thought that a new baby, a new chapter, would be the thing to put our marriage back on an even keel.

We were going through the motions of sex without birth control, but I don't think either of us really thought that we'd get pregnant. We certainly weren't thinking properly about what would happen if we did. In the event, when that second line did appear on the test, I was ecstatic. Bryn was ambivalent, which upset me more than I thought it would.

The thing is, the only reason I'd done the test was because I had been bleeding on and off for a month. I hadn't been worried. My periods had always been patchy and irregular, different lengths apart and varying in duration. The flow was usually fairly light but could sometimes be heavy. So for there to be this type of bleeding was a little unusual but didn't make me unduly anxious, especially because I wasn't experiencing any kind of pain.

When I finally called the doctor about it, he asked me several triage questions and at the end, almost to tick it off, said, "And could you be pregnant?" I laughed and said no. But of course, it made me reassess, and before I went in for a fast-track appointment the next day, I did a test. At the doctor's they double-confirmed my pregnancy and checked me over. Then they sent me straight off the same day to the hospital for more tests.

"Just in case", they kept saying. "It's just a precaution." But underneath the bright smiles and brisk efficiency, there's always a hint of the worry. I remember being bright at first too, but I also remember my depression (it was bad at that time) and the tears soaking my face. I tried to talk myself into calm, held it together on the surface and followed the instructions pragmatically. Just do this next thing. It was one of those whirlwind days where you have to cancel or forget all the appointments and tasks you have in the diary. One of those ones where you finally get home in the evening to see your laptop is still open, sentences half-written, cold cup of tea half-drunk on the table, papers everywhere.

I went to the hospital and called Bryn on the way. I didn't know how long I would be there and with the NHS (to be clear, I adore it and we need to do more to fund its brilliant work) it's always best to prepare yourself for a long wait. It would be school pick-up time before long and we had to arrange cover. I think I cried because of the uncertainty of it all and because I needed support.

At the hospital they took bloods, scanned me, asked me questions over and over. With ectopic pregnancies you measure the increasing levels of hCG (human chorionic gonadotropin).[1] So after these blood samples were taken, I had to go back the next day for more so they could measure the difference in levels and work out how much the embryo was growing. This can indicate whether or not it's growing at the correct rate; when a pregnancy is ectopic, it's not.

They said they would call me the day after the second test to let me know the results. But I chased them and they discovered the second sample had been lost. So I went in late that day for take two (or three). They didn't lose it this time, but they still needed more data, so I went back again for another test that Sunday in the emergency room as well. Monday came around and with it a mid-morning phone call. "We need to see you again. Can you come this afternoon?"

I had an internal ultrasound, and they finally said the words I'd been preparing myself for. "I'm sorry, but I can see the embryo in the fallopian tube. I just need to get a second opinion." From then it was a blur of swishing curtains, hospital beds, phone calls, ward admission and surgery that evening. I was lucky that it was caught before the embryo grew too big and burst my fallopian tube. When this happens, women can lose a lot of blood and sometimes even die.

The whole experience was surreal, and happened so swiftly that sometimes it's hard to compute how I felt. I was in shock for a few days afterwards. And the thing about shock is that you don't really realise that you're experiencing it. I found myself weeping one day on the floor of the shower after I removed the tiny little plasters covering my keyhole surgery scars. It didn't hurt, and I'd recovered well. But the tears came on me like a wave and I felt faint.

I like to think of myself as a no-nonsense, independent woman, but I was shocked in a way by my body's reaction. For once I leant into this and the support that Bryn gave me. We'd been spitting divorce at each other at the time, and in a way (for me at least) the pregnancy loss scared us into realising what we meant to each other. They tell you you have to hit rock bottom to come up to the top again: that's what that moment felt like to me.

It prompted a whole reassessment of our marriage, lives and goals, as well as my mental health and how we were impacting each other. We had piles of therapy. Decided what we really wanted and what would make us stronger in the longer term. We moved back to London. But were we ready to get back on the horse again with another child after that loss? That took us longer to determine.

Our therapist suggested a trial period. A sort of test – to force us to really find out if being together was the best thing for us and our daughter. We should test the waters of our new intentions with a year of living back in London. We didn't buy a house, but rented one for that year: it was part of the trial and would take the pressure off us. Because we took the pressure off, sex actually felt more comfortable. Intimacy still had its ups and downs at times (whose doesn't when you're grown-ups with responsibilities and time pressures?) but we were able to enjoy ourselves and our bodies more freely, without the thought that this might be make or break for our marriage. And without worrying about whether we would or wouldn't get pregnant. So I felt only joy when after a few months back in London we found ourselves wanting to take the next step and try for another baby again. It felt right. The day we moved into the new house we'd bought after our trial year, I found out I was pregnant.

The Word on the Street

Rosalie Genay, singer/songwriter, mum of two

"[The effects of sexual assault] have been so hush-hush for such a long time. Talking to other people, I've found that so many people have their own stories and things that they're still carrying with them. People are not really paying attention and there's no space to process it either. If there is space, you're not being supported in that process.

With my first pregnancy, I felt like people saw me and even wanted to touch me. As soon as the baby arrives, there is this massive shift; you become the invisible mother, while everyone focuses on the baby, yourself probably included.

I've experienced two pregnancies: one in the UK and one in the Netherlands. In the Netherlands, they did ask 'are there other any things that we need to be aware of, such as sexual assault or any experiences that you think might have an impact on your pregnancy or the check-ups?', which wasn't a feature for me in the UK.

When they asked me in Holland, I was there by myself and I actually felt like I needed to tell them but I didn't know if I could. It made me incredibly emotional, but I did end up giving a brief explanation of my experiences with sexual assault and previous birth trauma. But I also know from speaking to others that there might be situations in which you don't feel comfortable at that particular moment to share what is needed, for example if your partner who is there with you isn't aware of your history. It's nice to be asked in the maternity process, but I think it could be done in a more sensitive way, and followed up. It shouldn't be a form-filling exercise.

If you're in that situation, there needs to be a red flag whenever anyone opens up your file. Otherwise you still have to advocate for yourself whenever you have an appointment, or justify if you don't want a male midwife to give you a sweep or do an examination; you have to be really vocal about it. For the actual labour in the Netherlands, it's all rather clinical: 'These are the rules.' For example, if you've had a caesarean before, you're not allowed to give birth anywhere else other than under medical supervision in a hospital. It's not entirely true, but that's how it's presented. You could say no, but then basically they're saying, well, if anything goes wrong, it's on you. And there is still the archaic thinking that you have to be on your back to give birth because it's easier for [medical staff]. Or there's a really high percentage of episiotomies. I found all of this quite difficult to manage, as it reminded me of my lack of autonomy during the rape.

In terms of rehabilitation after birth and sex after birth, I did see a pelvic floor specialist who helped with the physical symptoms after the first birth, and then I had one therapy session too. At the time I thought, 'I can't actually do this: it's too much.' But then when I was pregnant the second time around, I started feeling really anxious about what was going to happen with the birth, and I thought I need to do something about it at this point, because otherwise there won't be a healthy way of going into it.

One of the midwives at my hospital was also a coach for prenatal women. So I saw her and then I had a few systems in place to feel more positive and plan out the pre-birth. The birth wasn't great, but then post-birth, it all started going wrong. Physically it was quite difficult; I had a lot of pelvic floor issues, and I couldn't really walk and stand properly. My husband was back travelling after two weeks too. I was alone most of the time with a toddler and a newborn, in a place where I didn't really know anyone. That's when things got pretty bad psychologically; I started feeling like I couldn't cope.

So I looked up a counsellor who dealt with issues such as historical sexual abuse but also did a lot of work with mothers. I went to the GP here in the Netherlands, too, to say I needed to see someone and, amazingly, the referral was instant. The next day I could see someone. I had tried to do this in the UK and it was six months before I was even called for a first appointment. I know that there is an enormous amount of privilege there. I really appreciate that. I do believe that it's saved me, because I don't know where I'd be otherwise.

I've always thought of myself as rather rational and sensible, and quite a calm person. And I struggled with being so overcome by something that I wasn't in control of, and how long the effects of the rape lasted. Being confronted with something you thought you had successfully pushed away for so long, it's really scary. And when you're a mother, too, having to deal with all of this and also having to care for other people at the same time . . .

You feel embarrassed and you feel like you should know better and that you should be better at coping.

I've always been someone who says 'I'll just deal with it.' To realise that actually you're not fine and you can't figure it out by yourself anymore, that's really strange.

Over the course of a year I had quite a few sessions with the psychologist, I had EMDR therapy and I also had group counselling, with women who were all dealing with their own similar things. It's not just about processing what's happened – it's also about looking forward. And for me, it was really important that I dealt with everything so I could avoid passing all that stuff on to my children. I had found it really difficult to regulate myself at times; I was easily triggered by certain things.

I wouldn't have been able to move on without the therapy. I also think it's almost impossible for a partner to understand what's going on, and it was too much for him to carry on his own. He has been really supportive and it must have been quite scary for him to see the person that he loves going through something like that. Because he was away so much, maybe he didn't initially fully grasp how bad it was, either – I think most women are good at making do.

After the rape, I had a really strange relationship with sex. If I was in charge, I could probably do it most of the time, but it took me years to lie on my back and be able to have intercourse in that way. And every now and then I would have an association and would not be able to continue, but that was pretty rare. So I suppose that's why I thought I was fine. And I could definitely enjoy sex. I think sex is really important and it can be amazing fun, and it *should* be fun.

Now, after my second child, I've had pelvic floor therapy again, and sex is kind of good. We're definitely more tired and have less time alone, so it can feel more of an effort to instigate sex! Often I'm not in the same country as my husband either, which doesn't help. But we have a much more open line of communication about those things now – if I'm not in the right headspace, or if I happen to switch off halfway through, I can just say that. And it's fine.

[Trauma and life-stage changes] are where a lot of relationships are probably broken or lost because the talking stops and the work stops. The entire conversation [about relationships after kids], not just about trauma, but the whole conversation, just needs to be more open. It really makes such a big change to women's lives. It's sad if we normalise our experiences and act like they're not important. It's important that we can talk about it, and hopefully that will also mean that healthcare and other systems will begin to work in our favour. We're in danger of losing a lot of women in society, because they're not fully functioning or happy. At the moment we don't help women after childbirth, when they feel at their most vulnerable and they need help the most."

What to Do Now

This might have been a tough chapter for you to navigate. Please do seek expert advice to help you work through what might be some powerful feelings. Therapy and medication are nothing to be ashamed of; in fact, we should be proud of ourselves for reaching out for help when we need it. That is an incredibly brave thing to do.

If you are looking for further help and information, the first thing to do is see your GP. It's not always easy to get an appointment, or even attend an appointment when you have a baby in tow, but I know you have the courage and clarity to advocate for yourself. The sooner you see your GP, the sooner you can ask for a referral to further mental health services (especially as this can take some time) and access medication if you feel that's right for you. If you are able to access services privately, this can be an extremely effective way forward too, and a much quicker one.

Talking therapy can be an absolute game-changer, as you'll know from my story and those of other experts who feature in the book. They can get you to where you want or need to be, even if it seems a really long way away. Or they can help you make peace with where you are now. Or both. How do you know you're ready? If what you're going through is "bad" enough? I used to ask myself this all the time. Growing up, I had the impression that therapy was for extreme issues. People on the edge. That if I had therapy I would be classed as some kind of nutjob too. But, as I slowly came to realise, the fact is, it's for anyone who feels it will make a difference. It's for you if where you are is not sustainable or healthy. And to be honest, that's most of us at one point or another. I now think therapy is fine. More than fine. It's brilliant. So if you're wondering . . . why not give it a go? It can't hurt to try, can it?

Get Your Mojo Back 101

Dr Alexandra Kasozi, clinical psychotherapist @the_psyched_mama

"Mental health, and particularly birth trauma, or any trauma, can of course impact intimacy. For example, let's say you've had a traumatic birth and that part of the experience for you was not feeling listened to. Perhaps you had a lot of people crowded around you, particularly while lying down and defenceless, perhaps you didn't feel you'd given consent for vaginal checks, or perhaps you experienced disempowering language. Even if you have no experience of previous sexual trauma, these experiences in a birthing situation can then potentially influence how you feel about your body in intimacy. Giving birth is an incredibly intimate thing to do. Ideally, what our mammalian brains would love is for us to be giving birth in the dark on our own or with our closest companions. And no one interfering with your vagina without permission, and having a completely safe space. The conditions under which you would ideally give birth and those under which you would have sex are actually quite similar. So if you've had a traumatic birth and those conditions haven't been present, either mentally or contextually, and you've been left feeling vulnerable, exposed or in danger at this highly intimate time, then having sex can be incredibly triggering for you.

Birth is a physiological event. But we know that the mind and body are intrinsically linked. How we are spoken to, and whether or not what others say and how they act make us feel safe can influence our body's ability to birth. Language matters. With birth, you can't get up and run away and you can't fight aggressors, so having people that feel like your protectors around you, people that are there for you and taking care of you, is important. Research shows us that feeling unsafe, feeling powerless and not feeling listened to are commonly reported factors when birthing people have experienced a traumatic birth or have PTSD related to childbirth.[2]

You're exposing yourself again with your partner and becoming vulnerable again. Often with a body that doesn't necessarily feel like your own. It's certainly not the body that you had before birth, even if it feels roughly the same. It's functioning differently, and it has a new meaning, so reconciling that, if you had a traumatic birth, or another traumatic experience prior to birth, it can be difficult."

What Next?

If you're not ready for outside help or you're still processing, there's lots you can do for yourself, too.

- **Talking:** My old favourite, yes. But yes, I will be harping on about it again, for all the reasons I've talked about before. The prime one being that you know how you're feeling and it's obvious to you why you're behaving a certain way, but it might not be obvious to your partner, even if they were beside you the whole way. I experienced exactly this with Bryn and the impact of my birth trauma; it was astonishing to me that he didn't get it, but equally it was a marker of how badly we had been communicating.
- **Be honest with yourself:** It's important to own how you're feeling, but it's just as important to be able to communicate that with your other half. Don't try to hide or pretend you're okay if you're not. It's okay to be struggling – the things we go through can be enormous.
- **Take time for you:** Some of this stuff can be hard to process when we're bogged down in the everyday stuff of parenthood and life. When we're feeling all touched out or in desperate need of some space, it's difficult to make the time for any mental clarity. Even going for a walk every other day on your own, drinking a coffee by yourself, reading a book or meditating can be helpful to build self-compassion and lead to a clearer headspace for you to think things through when you're ready..

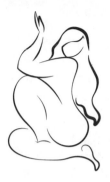

THE FUN STUFF

Enjoying intimacy and getting passionate again.

Phew! I hope that although this book deals with a lot of issues, you've felt unburdened after reading about my story as well as others' experiences, plus felt empowered by the wisdom of some truly amazing experts. I hope you've learned about how to resolve those issues and get your mojo back, even just a little bit.

Somehow things seem to take on a serious tone when we become parents (adulting can be hella boring). So now: lucky you! In this chapter there's a whole HEAP of fun stuff! Okay, you might have solved your pain or numbness. We might have started to clear your head of trauma or depression, and set you on the path to actually wanting to have sex again. We may even have taught you how to think about making the time for some booty-loving . . . but what if you're just not feeling inspired any more? What if you're turned on by different stuff these days? What if you just need a bit more of a boost to rock each other's worlds these days? You know, now that you've been together for a while and there's the small matter of having created a small human together.

Sex, like your relationship itself, is a journey. We change as we grow – as individuals, and together as a couple. When that relationship goes through a milestone like becoming parents . . . well, there's a reason you feel such a shift. It's a completely different life stage and you're entering a brand new phase of your relationship. The connection you have always had will be tested and stretched. You might grow distant, and you'll certainly need to make an effort to talk to each other every once in a while.

So, here I'm going to talk about low pressure, fun and (above all) realistic ways to get to know yourself and each other again. From learning what you are comfortable with now and whether you're turned on by the same things (as your pre-birth self or as each other), to figuring out which wands might be the ones to sprinkle some magic into your bed. Sex is a deep connection, and it's supposed to spark joy. Or you're supposed to at least halfway enjoy it. So this chapter is about setting you on the road to achieving that again. It might seem impossible, but it doesn't have to be.

This chapter isn't supposed to guilt you into sex if you're not ready. Quite the contrary. Remember what I've said about us all being different and our journeys being unique. This chapter is here for when you *are* ready. But it might also serve to get your imagination going if you're not quite there yet. Sometimes we can forget about how good sex is and what we liked about it in the first place. And if that's you, and you need a little reminder, then I reckon you'll find this bit of the book pretty helpful too.

Finding the Light at the End of the Tunnel

Yeah, yeah, I know, it's cheesy. But there really is a happy ending to my story. I suffered a pretty comprehensive catalogue of postnatal difficulties, both physical and mental. To say our relationship and my self-esteem suffered is an understatement. We didn't just lack warmth and intimacy, we were in a desert in the middle of the night.

But I got through it. I found shit out, I advocated for myself, I kept asking questions and I did the rehab and (groan) self-care.

When I re-tell it, it sounds straightforward; with the benefit of hindsight, things often do. But in reality it was a mess. It was not a linear journey. Improvement wasn't easy. And I'm one of the lucky ones. I had the support of my husband; I'm also privileged in that I had the time and intelligence to do my own research and seek out experts. I was so unhappy that I felt compelled to be persistent. So, yes, it was a long journey, but our sex life is now positive, fun-filled, satisfying and, thank god, pain-free. Hip, hip, hooray!

My Story

Although we would still have some big relationship stuff to deal with later, when I started to come out of my first couple of years of postnatal recovery, I began to feel hopeful again about sex. There was so much relief that I might finally be seeing the results of my physical rehabilitation work. I went from yearning and "don't touch me" vibes in equal amounts, to actually feeling like sex could be an enjoyable part of our lives again.

While the first year after my daughter was born was spent trying to figure out what the hell was going on, the second year felt more positive, more hopeful. I used to think that first year was a year wasted, and was frustrated by the length of time it had taken to get to an answer, but I now recognise that if I hadn't been through it, I wouldn't be nearly so passionate about the cause now, and you wouldn't be reading this book!

Year two's rehab saw me work on my hypertonic pelvic floor to bring flexibility and mobility to my muscles, using focused relaxation, stretches and balancing out the other areas of tightness in my body. Reader, you might not be surprised to hear that these areas were pretty much all over – I was so wound up and stressed that my entire body was tense. I continued to work on my episiotomy and vaginal scar desensitisation, and I *really* worked on being less scared and more present in sex, so that I wasn't inadvertently seizing up for penetration. All of this focused physical work would set the scene for the following years of personal development, which would be more concentrated on my mental health, trauma reactions, depression and rage.

During that second year, and especially toward the end of it, I began to feel stirrings of an interest in intimacy again. Making lurve (cue Barry White) was back on the agenda. Or was it? I was interested in exploring again, and had had enough of feeling disconnected as a couple and less than whole as a woman. As the pain reduced and I became more forgiving of my body and my trauma, I started to be able to relax properly again. Recovery is rarely a linear journey, and there were still moments, of course, when I wanted to stop, when things didn't feel right. These were points when I was too wound up to allow my mind to help me relax; my hypertonic pelvic floor would become even more hyper, instead of responding to all the release work I'd been doing.

One thing I really struggled with was understanding, and being comfortable with, the role that my body had to play in my identity now. A lot of my tension was due to the stress of new motherhood, sure, but it was also because I just couldn't marry up the dual roles of my vagina: a child-bearing vessel and an object of sexual pleasure. And it took a long time to change the narrative in my head. Just when I thought I had a handle on it, a thought or flashback would whistle into my head to stop us in our tracks. As time went on and the grip of the birth trauma loosened, things improved. And with more time, as I rehabilitated my body, I felt stronger and more confident in it again. I felt a little more in control as the confusion of new motherhood gave way, slowly, to clarity. I felt like I was on the way to the person

I should be, which meant that my identity got a boost and in turn intimacy felt more positive and loving.

But, as you may have noticed, a lot happens to our bodies through pregnancy, birth and postnatally. So what did that mean for my body and the things that turned me on? Were they the same? We'll all be different, so this might not be your experience, but I found that some things were heightened and some were muted. It meant that while overall the sex we'd always had was good enough, we also had to explore new ways of being together, both from a practical point of view and mentally.

For the sake of my painful vagina, which I'd spent so long working on, we had to make adjustments to penetrative sex. Firstly, and probably unsurprisingly, we did less of it. Then, when I was eventually more comfortable with it, we took it slowly; if I felt out of kilter, we stopped before we would have done before; we adjusted speed and rhythm; we played around with new positions that would be comfortable for me; and around all of that, we focused way more on things other than penetration. We massaged, we teased, we kissed and cuddled; and incredibly, it all added up to a much more intimate experience than we'd probably expected. Some of these things are not what we've been led to believe add up to hot sex: kissing and touching are portrayed as boring, or as the lead-up to "the real thing" – or they're simply not portrayed at all. But if that's how you've been taught too, you might be in for a pleasant surprise. Those multitudes of intimate touches and gestures added up not just to romance, but to heightened awareness, sensitive reactions and a slow-building arousal, and it really paid off in the end.

We didn't go into this wanting to cut out penetration completely, and I think if you'd asked us then, we might not have thought the changes we incorporated would be long-term. But the things we explored added another dimension to our sex life which has brought a depth of flavour that we wouldn't have otherwise. We added some (apologies to all the non-foodies out there) umami, if you will. And you know what? It was so good, we've kept it.

The restriction on PIV (penis-in-vagina) sex meant that we were forced to become more creative, and, while it sounds so obvious, it could have easily gone the other way. At times it did: when it just didn't feel "worth it" to have sex if it wasn't about penetration. I'm glad that we persevered with intimacy when we could. Because for me (and of course we're not all the same) sexuality and sensuality is an important part of a relationship or marriage, one that I'm not willing to forego. Of course there are a fair number of other reasons that Bryn and I are together! But intimacy definitely completes the package.

When I look back on that period now, I think it was an obvious move to make, tweaking and altering our sex lives to make it better for both of us, but it's surprising how many of us don't do that. We might feel awkward about it, so we don't stop to analyse it for ourselves; if we're not really aware of it, then we don't bring it up with our partners. Then, because we're not talking about it, we might not realise the other is dissatisfied. And so it goes on. What a vicious circle.

Well, huzzah, now we were getting onto more of an even keel, I actually felt like having sex a bit more. I can't tell you how much of a relief that was. I've always thought that sex begets sex: one suggested way of relighting your relationship fire is to have sex every night (or day) for a month, the theory being that you'll want to have more sex afterwards. We didn't go that far, but I did find that once you've had a taste, you remember how enjoyable sex can be. It would linger in our minds and mean that we were more likely to go again.

As we felt more turned on by each other and the thought of being together, we felt freer to explore. We were more honest with each other about what we liked and didn't like, we talked dirty during sex (yes, it is awkward at the beginning and yes, it does get better, quickly), we went free range and roamed (say what now?) outside the bed. We listened to audio-erotica alone and together, we explored porn that we both felt comfortable with, we got some decent toys that were beautiful as well as sexy, there were even blindfolds and knots involved at times. This might be old hat to you; it is to me now. It might be all new and a little bit tantalising. Or it might be new and not up your street at all. In any case, there is a special frisson about trying something new that rejuvenated our sex life, and learning it together was an added bonus. Bryn was not my first sexual rodeo and I wasn't his. So getting to know each other in new ways, being vulnerable again and putting trust in each other, listening and learning together was actually incredibly bonding, whether we ended up loving what we tried or not.

Over the course of several months and years, it was a smorgasbord of sensuality. Some stuff worked and some didn't. We kept bits and let some go. But the point is that we tried them. Sometimes (as is usually the case the first time you do something) it felt embarrassing, but knowing that one or other, or both, of us wanted to try it made sure we kept an open mind. If you're on the same page, know where your boundaries are and you can avoid taking yourself too seriously, it's a really great starting point. And you know what? We had a giggle, and we enjoyed ourselves, whether we ended up discovering our new favourite sexy-time thing or not. Sex is sexy, sure. It's sensual, slow and passionate. But it should also be fun, and pleasure doesn't have to be serious. Laughing breaks tension, and also releases endorphins, which all contribute to the good times.

Try something more than once, and whatever that new thing is might suddenly turn out to be revolutionary.

The thought of us getting to experiment with all of this would have seemed impossible just a year earlier. We needed to feel comfortable with each other, and to actively want to support one another too. Both of us, and me in particular, also needed to be at ease with ourselves and open to sharing what we wanted. While there were things that we still needed to work on (remember that divorce we almost had?), we were at least back to connecting in a meaningful way sexually, and my gosh, what a difference that made.

It Starts with Me

So often we get the message from books, films and TV that sex is about getting it on with another person. Or more than one other person. But what about the first person you should be getting to know? You know me well enough by now: I'm talking, of course, about yourself.

Yes, this book is about rehabilitation and relationships, making love and making it work with your partner, but like many a good pop song will tell you, it starts with you. I'm talking about the (wo)man in the mirror. This is about you first. If you're not comfortable with yourself, if you don't know what you want, how on earth are you going to communicate it with someone else?

There's a serious lack of desire to educate women about female pleasure and feeling at home in your body. You know, I realised only after I had children that I never thought that my body was my own. The only thing I was interested in in terms of how I looked and whether I was sexy, was whether it was attractive to other people. I saw myself through the eyes of other people, never through my own eyes.

Natalie Lee, Author of **Feeling Myself**

So, let's start this journey by getting curious. When was the last time you properly got to know yourself? Explored and found what made you tick? Discovered the pleasure of an orgasm? I'm betting it was in your adolescence. As your body grew and changed, you sprouted hair and your breasts swelled. Those changes sound surprisingly similar to the changes of pregnancy, don't they? So perhaps it's not such a surprise after all that we need to get to know ourselves again after this big transformation too.

We are often taught to view ourselves and our pleasure through the lens of others. When we're in adolescence and early adulthood, this tends to be through the lens of potential partners – for many of us (as women), this is, therefore, through the male gaze. We end up thinking that other people's opinions are the ones that count, not our own. We judge our bodies by whether they are pleasing to others, not whether *we* like them. We dress to impress others, we choose clothes based on the latest fashions, whether they suit us or not, and we end up caring entirely *too much* about what we look like. We learn about blow jobs and penetration before we even know where our clitoris is. In most countries we're taught that sex is for making babies, and learn nothing about the role it plays in pleasure and fulfilment. We are taught about the mechanics but not the emotions. We aren't encouraged to explore or take ownership of our own bodies. The superb Hollie McNish has a fantastic poem on this called "Conversations with Kids",[1] referring to PIV sex as "the only type of sex they'll teach you all to count". Based on my experience, that seems pretty fair.

Get Your Mojo Back 101

Sophie Whippy, sex educator and doula @_sophiewhippy

"Countless people now in their thirties, forties, plus are either at a point where they are waking up to the possibilities of actually being allowed to take ownership of a fulfilling sex life, or they are at such a point of disconnect that their sex life is the least of their concerns. Conditioning starts when we're young, when we absorb all the patterns we see, like our parents' intimacy, or hearing lewd jokes and awkwardness around sex. Then we hit school. The RSHE [relationships, sex and health education] curriculum was updated in 2019 – the first review since 2000, and although updates are always welcome, there are still missing pieces. In a recent survey by the Sex Education Forum, 46 per cent of young people said the topic of pleasure wasn't even addressed and only one in five young people felt there was time to ask questions.[2]

Female sexuality and pleasure is still possibly one of the most taboo subjects, with sex being approached in popular culture, media, mainstream literature, all from the male gaze perspective. Women are held to different standards than men and always have been in many areas of life. This, combined with the gaping hole in school-taught sex education and the patriarchal oppression of women being disempowered historically, that leads us to where we are now – many women not feeling comfortable with their own physicality.

A postpartum body is in hormonal flux, and a new parent is learning and often emotionally exhausted; this of course can have huge effects on how intimacy is explored. I believe the key to rebuilding or discovering new ways to explore intimacy is to communicate. Open, continuous, verbal communication is paramount in keeping both

> parents working together, and avoids isolating one from the other. People feel safe and seen when they are heard. Truly listening is a skill and one that needs practising; learning how to do this in a relationship can be the biggest asset to your intimate life."

In traditional school curricula, and in Western society, we aren't taught to nurture our own self-love or freedom in our bodies. As women, we don't tend to our own pleasure nearly as much as we tend to that of others. And I'm not just talking about our sexual partners. When you become pregnant, your body is taken over by something – someone – else. Suddenly you're watching what you eat, feeling different, abstaining from caffeine or alcohol, experiencing changing emotions and nausea, literally walking through the world in an entirely new and different way. Then afterwards, when we become a parent, particularly a mother, we spend so much of our time putting our needs second. What ends up mattering is the baby, the kids, the chores, the juggle, rather than what we want and need.

Intimacy and sexual pleasure barely feature, and often we end up dissatisfied with ourselves because we think that our needs are less important than the needs and desires of others. Perhaps now is the time to redress the balance. You're at a big life-stage change, so why not take advantage of it? It's a time of change, and a time of newness. Rediscovery is the name of the game.

Self-Pleasure Isn't Selfish

Building up confidence anew by exploring your body and your boundaries is a great place to start. I talked a little about masturbation in Chapter 4; whether that's newly postnatally or further down the motherhood line, taking time to understand yourself and what turns you on, without the pressure of another person, can be the key to unlocking yourself again (or maybe for the first time).

Your body may have changed; it might feel different to touch and to be in and react differently to the same prompts. It's hard to articulate these changes to your partner if you're not even sure what they are yourself. So it's worth taking the time to establish where you are now, if you feel differently, if you're turned on in different ways. Explore yourself. Masturbate. Ask yourself: what kind of touch is pleasurable? How much time does it take to turn myself on? Is slower/quicker better? Do I want to avoid certain things? Are parts of my body ready for this?

It might feel selfish, but literally taking the time to be by yourself and tune into your body and needs could be just the thing you need. If it feels weird to hole up in the bedroom while your partner is elsewhere, take a bath and do it there. If even that feels too much, steal a few minutes in the shower, or while you're getting changed. If it does feel overwhelming, what might that mean for you and intimacy right now? Whatever you're feeling isn't wrong, it's just where you are. Meet yourself there and let that be your jumping-off point, whether that's right back where you left off before pregnancy or somewhere completely different.

Alternatives to Sex

When most people think of sex, they think of PIV sex. Statistics vary, but only around 25 per cent of women experience orgasm from penetration alone.[3] The clitoral tissue extends way beyond the visible nub (glans) we usually refer to as the clitoris, which means that actually the clitoris is involved in penetrative sex too; however, most of us probably find that some focus on the clitoris (glans) by itself wouldn't go amiss either.

So. Traditional penetrative sex. Well, that's great and all, but why not focus on the other stuff for once? This is a particularly good idea after birth or in rediscovering ourselves. Physical and mental trauma and rehab might mean that you're just not ready yet for penetration. Or you are and you're not finding it pleasurable, or you're just not feeling anything at all. If PIV sex is just not floating your boat, there's so much other stuff you can try instead. The best thing is that taking penetration off the table takes the pressure off the whole act of intimacy, and in indulging in things like kissing and touch alone, you'll probably find that you're left wanting more. It might just be a great way to kick off that slow burn back to desire that you've been looking for.

So yes, I'm singing from the rooftops about the virtues of kissing, non-penetrative options, intimacy without sex and how to cultivate romance without the pressure for intercourse. It might sound easy, but don't worry if you find it a bit "meh" at first, especially if you haven't really done it since you were a teen in your parents' living room. Persevere, and it can be really beautiful and a huge turn on to just take penetration off the table for a while. Plus, if you're wondering, it definitely doesn't mean that orgasms are out of the question too.

- **Kissing:** An oldie but a goodie. Make time for an old-fashioned tongue twister, a snog on the sofa, whether you're pretending to watch a movie or not. We can often become complacent in our kissing, and get used to the way our partners do it. Why not change it up? Mix techniques and speed, use soft biting. Kiss other bits of the face, play around with the position of your faces. Add in some anticipation and delay contact. When you focus on the basics, you can find that they're actually much more of a turn on than you realise.
- **Getting handsy:** Another teen fave that can actually be startlingly sexy. Sure, a fumble or a grope is probably not top of your list of sophisticated moves, but again, slowing it down, experimenting with different pressures and types of touch can build delicious tension. If you're stopping here, or after kissing, hopefully a touch of sexy suspense will help reignite your desire for next time too.
- **Cunnilingus and fellatio:** These can be so much more special than the names "blow job" or "going down on someone" imply. Take time to figure out what you both like

now, because if you haven't checked for a while, it might well be different to what you have been doing! Slow it down, experiment with timing, pressure, different areas of the vulva and penis. Throw in an exploratory hand if you like, too. Now is a good time to add in lube (make sureit's organic!), especially if you haven't played around with it before and you want to get familiar with it before using it with penetration.

- **Intimacy without sex:** Or as some might see it, good ol' romance. Why not hold hands occasionally (when there's not a kid in between you), cop a cheeky feel as you pass in the kitchen, sit with each other, touching a part of their body you wouldn't normally – like the tops of thighs, the skin underneath your tee-shirt, the base of your neck. You might not be into touch right now, and if you need some space, that's also fine (see Chapters 3 and 4) but these ideas are great if you've had that space and want to reconnect.

Intimacy Aids

I don't know about you, but when I was growing up, the imagery that came to mind when I thought of dildos and vibrators was not entirely appealing. Scary-looking, too long and large, weirdly coloured and overly veiny, they didn't exactly scream a big friendly hello. The Rabbit came around, I can still remember the joyous breakthrough of Charlotte's *Sex and the City* obsession (if you know, you know), and suddenly there was a new, more welcoming, bunny-eared face of sex toys. I'm not suggesting that you throw yourself headlong into Ann Summers (in fact, as you'll read, there are plenty of better options out there). And you don't have to get yourself on the invite list to a swinging party (unless you want to), but a good vibrator is just the tip of the iceberg. If you think you'll prefer vanilla, then you absolutely have my support. If you fancy trying out a bit of tutti frutti, there are plenty of options to choose from. And if you want to just upgrade your vanilla from kids' fave own-brand to artisanal gelato, there are options for you too.

Lube (Again) and Condoms

I'll champion sexual lubricant until the cows come home, because it's nothing to be ashamed of, will make things much more pleasurable and will mean you're not damaging the sensitive tissues of your amazing body if dryness is a problem for you. Get an organic one (my favourite is YES Organics), and get one now. Make sure you choose the water-based option if you're using condoms; oil-based lube has a thicker feel and is suitable for non-condom sex. The right condoms are another quick win. Choose an eco friendly brand with fewer/no chemicals that is less likely to irriatate; these are usually beautifully branded too – so if you have a choice, you might as well! Hanx is a good place to start.

Sex Toys

Female-curated and female-designed sex toys are now par for the course. They look beautiful and are pleasing colours; some can easily pass for an *objet d'art* if you leave them out on display. And they feel great; shaped with us in mind, they're also usually made with non-irritating materials – a far cry from the tacky plastic and sticky rubber of old. What's most interesting to me (and I don't know how it took so long for the makers to make this leap) is that they're now actually designed for women. That might sound obvious, but what I mean is that sex toys are now more, much more, than just a replica penis. Instead of designing through the male gaze, today's intimate brands are focusing on what we want to hold or feel, both on and in our bodies. Can our smaller hands hold them properly? Does it fit inside a handbag, if that's your jam? Does it stimulate the clitoris properly? Is it easy to wash? Can you adjust the vibrations so it's not an absolute racket? What I'm saying is that if you were worried about venturing into sex-toy territory before, it might be worth a revisit. I've listed a few friendly places to start in the resources at the end of the book.

Teases

But intimacy aids aren't just about that kind of toy. You might find now is the time to explore fantasies that you've long held but haven't acted on. A little (or a lot, if that floats your boat) kinkiness never hurt anyone if you and your partner are on the same page. If you find you need something more to focus on to get you in the mood these days (I hear you), introducing something different could help draw your mind in. Or perhaps your body and senses have changed and you just want those extra stimuli. Maybe the build-up needs to be longer and you need something to fill the gap. Whatever it is, it's okay to give it a go. Some starters for ten:

- **Use what you have:** Always fancied being tied up? Does a blindfold sound fun? It's amazing how useful a silk scarf can be. You can also use it to trail over the body and connect with the lesser-used erogenous zones.
- **Sexy undies:** I'm not talking about those cliched red, lacy (and uncomfortable!) sets from the nineties, unless that turns you on. What do you feel comfortable in or what makes you feel good? What shows you in the light you want to be seen? If you can't or don't want to spend money, that's totally fine – how can you rework what you have? We've usually got a halfway decent set hiding in the drawer. Remember that a tank top and boy pants can be equally alluring when worn with a plomb too! Often sex as parents is about diving into bed and having a quick tussle under the duvet. Perhaps taking time to slowly undress one another and appreciate each others' bodies will add a novelty to intimacy that you didn't realise you'd missed.
- **Massage!** An oldie but a goodie: sometimes we forget how good it is to let someone else do the work. It will relax you and get you reacquainted with simple feelings of pleasure again. Use oils that nourish your skin and it's a win-win. YES Organics oil-based lube (not for use with condoms) is made with coconut oil and perfect for massaging, so you won't have to go rummaging for the tube when the time comes.
- **Candles** might seem cheesy, but they really help set the

scene. A scented one might even do the trick of helping you forget about those piles of washing to do in the corner. Bright overhead lights don't do anything to reawaken the primeval part of the brain that's usually in charge for sex, so there is a higher purpose for sexy low lighting. Massage candles, made from oil that can be melted and then used on the skin, kill two birds with one stone. Remember to let it cool for a bit once melted!

Stories

Bodice-ripping Mills & Boon this isn't. Getting your erotica fix has come a long way from seeking out passages in a well-thumbed *Lady Chatterley's Lover* as a teen. I love a good novel (erotic bent or not) as much as the next woman, but sometimes you want to skip to the good part too. There are now stories to suit all tastes, to read or have read to you. In paper, online or on an app.

Perhaps it might not seem so thrilling to read a passage together in bed before embarking on a bit of rumpy-pumpy, but you can use it in different ways: have a sneak peak when you're away from each other, listen on your way home to build up the anticipation, send each other cheeky excerpts that turn you on. Or if you need a quick boost and want some input, but watching porn isn't for you, listen to something together while you're getting into foreplay. Dipsea and Ferly are two brilliant apps, but see some other suggestions in the resources at the end of the book.

Films

Whether you've previously watched porn or not, you'll probably be in for a pleasant surprise when you take a look at some of the films that are out there these days. While I do choose to watch porn occasionally and think it has a great role to play in partner sex (again, if you're both on the same page) as well as solo pleasure, mainstream options leave me conflicted, and I'm sure some of you will feel the same. Which is why it's so brilliant to see many more ethical and feminist porn film-makers out there now. It means you're seeing people who actually enjoy what they're doing and aren't being taken advantage of.

In ethical porn, performers are paid well and aren't marginalised, and you're seeing storylines that involve more than purely repeated thrusting, exaggerated sex noises and violence-adjacent scenes. That is to say, it's a touch more nuanced than traditional porn. A good way to tell if it's feminist or ethical is to see whether any of the performers are also involved in producing or directing and whether it's paid for. Just do the same research you would in buying anything you care about – search out a bit of background about the film company and the people involved. There's so much on Google and social media, it's hard not to find the info that you need to make the right choice.

And yes, I know we're used to consuming so much content for free these days (including porn), but it really does make sense to pay for it. And once you have paid, you can watch it as many times as you like. That seems pretty fair to me.

Fantasies and Dirty Talk

I'm not suggesting you dive straight into masked swingers' parties, but we all have scenarios that turn us on more than others. Is now a good time to start exploring those with your partner? It doesn't have to be full on whips and chains; you could just start with a little suggestive talk in bed, a whisper or two in each others' ears during the evening. It might just take you out of yourself too, which helps in transitioning from parentland to sexy time and might give you a boost if you're not quite feeling the confidence you once did in your body through its changes.

These suggestions might seem way out there for you, or you might already be thinking "yawn". Either way, exploring where you are now and testing the waters of something new might just help reignite your confidence and passion once you are ready.

Contraception!

I haven't talked much about contraception in this book, because frankly that's usually the only thing you get talked through comprehensively in your postnatal and maternity care. "Do you want a coil inserted at the same time as your C-section? Would you prefer the implant or the injection? If you opt for the pill, make sure you're going to be taking it regularly, as it's easy to forget when you've got a new baby!" In my six-week postnatal check, the only question I was asked about myself was what contraception I wanted to start using.

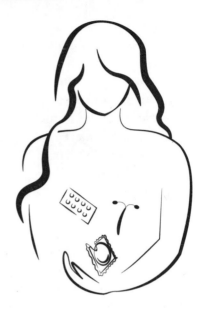

Finding the right contraception can often be key to enjoying postnatal sex (or any PIV sex), if you want to take away the potential worry of a pregnancy. It can also mean that once you're in the flow, there's less umm-ing and ah-ing about whether to continue, so it's a less stilted experience, especially if it's taken either or both of you a moment to find your pizazz again.

There will be many considerations, such as whether you can remember to take medication, whether your vagina gets irritated by synthetic materials inside it, if you are ready for the discomfort of fitting a coil, how you've previously reacted to contraceptive interventions (for example heavy bleeding) and how much you value convenience.

Maisie Hill's *Period Power* has a really excellent breakdown of contraceptive forms, both hormonally based and not, which I would definitely recommend reading. It's important to think about if you want to continue to use a hormonal contraceptive method or not, and to consider the effects it's had on you in the past (if you already have experience of one), as well as reading further into the impact that systematically taking synthetic hormones may have on your body long term.

Contraceptive options include:

- Temperature tracking and cycle timing
- Condoms
- Vasectomy for a man
- Sterilisation for a woman
- Contraceptive pill or mini-pill
- Contraceptive injection
- Contraceptive implant
- Hormonal coil
- Copper coil

The existence and continued promotion of hormonal contraception for women, developed in the main by men, is part of a larger feminist conversation around female bodily autonomy in a patriarchal tradition. Would the (sometimes severe) side effects of the pill be condoned if the pill were taken by men? The recent halting of development of the "male pill" due to just such side effects suggests not.[4] The onus has always been on women to prevent childbirth, despite the fact that (putting aside multiple births) men can father multiple children at any one point, whereas a woman can only be pregnant with one. I'm not saying I have the answer here, but after birth can be a really good time to reassess what your family plans are in the longer term, what you want to put into your body in the future and whether your partner might have a role to play in your contraceptive plans. The good news is that developments in new male contraception methods (such as an ultrasound testicle bath[5]) are making good progress.

I asked Dr Brooke Vandermolen to outline the vasectomy for me, as it's an option people rarely know much about. She says:

"A vasectomy (male sterilisation) is a surgical procedure to cut or seal the tubes that carry a man's sperm to permanently prevent pregnancy. It's usually carried out under local anaesthetic, where you're awake but don't feel any pain, and takes about 15 minutes. A vasectomy is more than 99 per cent effective. It's considered permanent, so once it's done you don't have to think about contraception again. It is possible to reverse, but this may not be successful, so vasectomy shouldn't be attempted if you aren't sure if your family is complete. It doesn't affect sex drive or ability to enjoy sex. Men can still have erections and ejaculate, but semen won't contain sperm. Some side effects of the procedure include bruising, swelling or pain in the ball sack (scrotum) – some men have ongoing pain in their testicles. As with any surgery, there's a small risk of infection."

Having the right contraception for you and being able to enjoy sex worry-free is a big part of fulfilling intimacy, so while it definitely shouldn't be the only thing we're asked about postnatally (less pressure, please!), do make sure you, both individually and as a couple, choose the best option in due course.

Couples' Therapy

It might sound dry, but it can help grease the wheels of conversation and help you understand what the other is going through. Once you like each other again, it's much more likely you'll want to have good sex with each other. Who'd have thought it, eh?

But look, I know it can seem like a big step. If you're on the verge of hating each other (or deep in the midst of it), please, just take the leap. It's nothing to be ashamed of. I can guarantee you that at least one of your sets of friends is doing it or has done it in the past. In the UK at least, we feel so much secrecy around talking therapy, particularly for relationships, but it is really one of the healthiest ways to make sure we're communicating properly.

If you think you're pretty much fine but something's just a bit off, that can also be a great reason to see someone. Or you can also use therapy as just a six-monthly or annual MOT to check in with each other and make sure you're on track. Too often when we're feeling a bit "meh", not engaging or feeling inexplicably annoyed by our partners, a neutral third party to help figure it out without all hell breaking loose is a really good idea.

If you can work out why you're annoyed by someone, it can help fix the issue. Which means you might like each other a bit more, be more attracted to your other half and even want to jump their bones on occasion too. Such is the circle of life. Some helpful hints for therapy? Read on!

- Don't write it off, thinking it's not for you. It doesn't just have to be for marriages on the verge of breakdown. Although obviously it's pretty useful for that too.
- Go in with an open mind. Whether you've done therapy before or not, each session is a chance to start anew. Use it to connect rather than get more entrenched in your position.
- Find the right therapist for you both. Sounds obvious, but having someone that both of you like is very helpful.
- Listen. Now, with a mediator, is the perfect time to let the other one have some airtime – and you'll get that opportunity too. Therapy is a safe and equal space.

Get Your Mojo Back 101

Lisa Williams, co-host of *The Hotbed* podcast and author of *More Orgasms Please* @lisa_of_the_suburbs

"It's important to find the right frequency and type of sex that works for you as an individual and as a couple. The standard idea of 'doing it' three times a week is one size that doesn't fit all. When you have little children, you can feel tired, 'touched out' from breastfeeding, carrying and cuddles, and stressed or anxious. Sex can often drop down the priority list. Equally, hormonal fluctuations can mean you feel like having lots of sex around the time of ovulation, and then none when you're pre-menstrual. But it all leads to the question of 'how do you define sex?' Will it always mean intercourse? Or both of you orgasming? Could it be solo sex as well as coupled? Or simply just a bit of fooling around? If you can adopt a looser definition, then the idea of frequency becomes much less urgent, and instead you can focus on connection, pleasure and relaxation.

Compared to many of our European counterparts, British women and mothers often struggle to express our desires and sensuality! I'd say that for every confident woman, there are at least 20 others who might be too embarrassed to voice their desires. We're conditioned to present ourselves as sexually attractive while remaining quiet about what we actually want. Not only that, but we often don't have the ideas, inspiration or the words to express ourselves, even if we want to.

Mainstream porn rarely features genuine female orgasms, and I grew up at a time when sex tips for women were things like, 'wear a push-up bra and give him a sexy tit-wank'. We sometimes don't know what we want and so we don't know what to say, and we might worry about hurting someone's feelings if we do speak out. I'm sure many women reading this have had awkward moments while a partner has tried to bring her to orgasm, feeling a mixture of embarrassment, shame and boredom . . . ! Many would rather fake it than say, 'Why don't we use some lube to get things going?' or 'I love what you're doing with your mouth but the nipple tweaking not so much . . .' Then, when we have children, we can often feel so embedded in the daily load of getting stuff done that we forget our sensual side; we may not have the money for nice underwear, vibrators and massage oil; at the end of the day, we might be so tired we just want to scroll through Instagram before passing out, and so on. Ironically, mutually pleasurable sex can be one of the most mindful and relaxing things you can do, but making the transition from mum life to sex life is a hurdle.

Finding headspace for sex in motherhood is all about finding a good 'gateway' activity that can transport you from feeling like a fraying dishcloth to a hot goddess. TV and social media aren't the best for this, as they don't energise you; instead, something like a bath, a brisk walk, a dance to your favourite music, even reading a book can be more relaxing and transitional than sticking on the TV after the kids' bedtime. Equally, putting pressure on yourself to have full-on sex can be a turn-off, so you could suggest a massage or a dance or cuddle in your underwear with no strings attached. These things will make you feel good and help you reconnect as a couple.

I definitely recommend trying toys or erotica. Both of these are a great shortcut to good sex for tired people, and can help you mix things up and experiment. And if you can, please pay for your porn, as you'll get a much better product; 'ethical porn' and 'real-life sex' such as Cindy Gallop's Make Love Not Porn platform will show you some hot scenes and get you in the mood or give you some ideas. As for sex toys, take your pick! Even those made from [more expensive] body-safe silicone are usually affordable and fun. Good ones to start with are clitoral stimulators such as the Womanizer, or you can move on to the full-on power of a 'wand' toy: try Sh! Women's Store for inspiration and advice.

What Next?

If you've never brightened up your sex life before, or never needed to (lucky you!), this chapter might seem a little overwhelming. It doesn't have to be. Treat this as a pick-and-mix trolley. Take what you want and leave what you don't. And if you try it and don't like it, choose a different candy next time. If and when you're interested in exploring further, check out the reading list and the other amazing resources at the back for more inspiration.

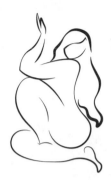

OVER AND OUT: CONCLUSION

Fly, my pretties!

Well, that was a tour and a half of some pretty juicy and important stuff. You might need to take a while to digest it. Go right ahead. You might want to jump straight in and solve some of those pressing issues. Yay! You might need more information. That's good too.

Wherever you find yourself, I hope this book has been a help, and at the very least a great starting point for your journey to wonderful, fulfilling, passionate sex and intimacy, whether that's with yourself or someone else. My goal in life is to make us (regardless of our gender) appreciate the importance of women's health and love ourselves just that little bit more, and just by reading this book, you've taken a hefty step in that direction – thank you.

If you have more questions or need more guidance, check out the (all together now) Resources that follow (including a decision tree for knowing where to start), the website for this book www.andbreathewellbeing.com/get-your-mojo-back or get in touch on Instagram @andbreathewellbeing.

Big hugs and more,

Clio x

Does it hurt when you have penetrative sex?

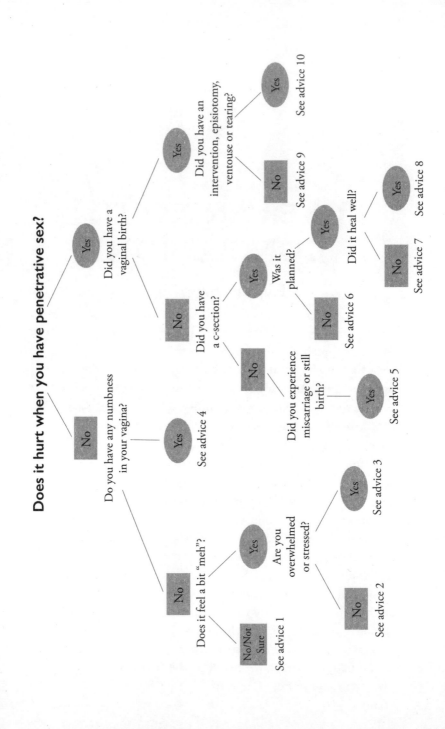

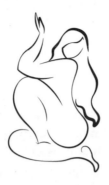

THE DECISION TREE!

Look, this whole book has contained a lot of information. And I know that for some you, especially, if it's all new info, it might seem like a minefield. So where on earth do you start? When you're not sure what the problem is, or when you have multiple issues, it can be hard to know how to go about finding an answer. The simplest thing to do is start with the easy stuff. Check and solve the quick wins, and you might find you're home free. If not, you know you've ticked a number of things off the list and you can now concentrate on some of the knottier problems. This decision tree could be a good tool to help you know where to begin.

Advice 1: Explore how you're doing mentally. Even if it doesn't feel like you have a mental health issue, our sex lives can be massively impacted by how we're doing emotionally. Individual and couples therapy might be a route you want to explore eventually but it's a good idea to start by talking to your GP/doctor too.

Advice 2: Start by exploring your relationship basics. Are you communicating? Have you had a date night recently? Do you even feel warm toward each other? It might be hard to want to get intimate if you're not even sure you like them!

Advice 3: Try a date night or two to reconnect, but remember that time on your own can also be a brilliant way to lessen any feelings of overwhelm or stress. That should help your relationship when you come back together. Games and intimacy aids can also be a great way to kickstart the fire if you've forgotten exactly how nice sex can be.

Advice 4: Numbness can be caused by a number of things. It's often a question of nerve-endings coming back to life, so desensitisation touch and massage can be great, as well as reconnecting with your breathing and pelvic floor muscles through PF exercises. Taking the time to mentally reconnect with your pelvic area can also be a nice way of remembering that part of your body. Talk to a women's health physio for more exercises and massage techniques. You can also check out these videos: andbreathewellbeing.com/get-your-mojo-back.

Advice 5: Trauma can affect our bodies and minds in ways that are unexpected. The mind–body connection is strong! Give yourself time to heal, talk to your support network and/or partner and talk to your GP/doctor about whether therapy is an option for you.

Advice 6: Unplanned and emergency c-sections can take time to heal both mentally and physically. Take enough time to process (at least 6–12 weeks) and once the scar has healed you might want to see a women's health physio and/or therapist to work through any trauma.

Advice 7: Talk to your GP about how the scar is healing both on the surface and in deeper layers. A women's health physio (don't be afraid to advocate for yourself to get a referral if necessary) can really help to unpick the impact of the scar on the rest of your body and core/pelvic floor. You might also find these videos helpful: andbreathwellbeing.com/get-your-mojo-back.

Advice 8: Check the tension of your scar (both on the surface and underlying tissue) and see if it might be pulling tissue and muscles from elsewhere on your body. A women's health physio will be able to tell you more in a personal assessment. Processing the birth mentally can also make a big difference to releasing any tension we are holding inadvertently. Building up proper functional strength during your rehab journey is also important. Are you doing your pelvic floor exercises properly? Check out my videos for more: andbreathewellbeing.com/get-your-mojo-back.

Advice 9: Sometimes the bruising from birth can have more of an impact than we think. Give yourself time to heal and explore any tenderness gently by yourself before you try for penetration. Also think about what your pelvic floor strength/tension is like. A women's health physio and proper pelvic floor exercises can make a really big difference here.

Advice 10: Are the scars/grazing from this healing well? Have you given yourself enough time to heal? It's ok to take it slowly. If you feel it's taking too long to heal, do check with your GP/doctor and ask for a referral to a women's health physio or gynaecologist to see if they can assess further.

GLOSSARY

Bruising: The pooling of blood under the skin following a blow or impact due to broken blood vessels

Candidal overgrowth: Overproduction of candida (a type of yeast/fungus) which can lead to yeast/fungal infections on the skin or in the vagina. Can also cause urinary tract infections, though these are usually not difficult to treat

Clitoris: Women's sexual pleasure organ. Its tissue extends way beyond the visible nub, or glans, that sits at the top of the vulva

Cut: Deliberate or accidental incision of skin/tissue

Dyspareunia: The medical term for painful pentrative sexual intercourse, either during or after sex

EMDR therapy: Eye Movement Desensitisation and Reprocessing. A form of psychotherapy that helps you process and recover from past experiences affecting your mental health and wellbeing. It involves using side-to-side eye movements combined with talk therapy in a specific and structured format

Episiotomy: Cut to the opening of the vagina made during childbirth to ease the passage of the baby's head and avoid tearing of vaginal tissue

Fourth trimester: The first three months after birth, referencing the three trimesters that pregnancy is traditionally divided into: first trimester, 1–3 months; second trimester, 3–6 months; third trimester, 6–9 months

Graze: A scrape that breaks the surface of the skin/tissue

Labia: Vulval lips

Matrescence: The period of growing into the identity of motherhood, becoming a mother

Melasma: Also called chloasma or "pregnancy mask", these are patches of grey/brown skin usually on the face, caused by an over-production of melanin (skin pigmentation). More common in women, and particularly likely (surprise surprise) to develop during pregnancy, they may fade postnatally after a few months. Treatments are available

Perineum: The tissue between the opening of the vagina and the opening of the anus

Postnatal: "After birth" – technically referring to the baby, but in practice used interchangeably with "postpartum"

Postpartum: After birth, technically referring to the mother, in practice used interchangeably with "postnatal"

PTSD: Post-traumatic stress disorder. A mental health condition that's triggered by witnessing or experiencing a terrifying or traumatic event. Symptoms can include flashbacks, nightmares and severe anxiety, as well as uncontrollable thoughts about the event

Scar: The tissue generated to replace normal skin after a wound is healed

Scar massage: Massage of the scar tissue and area surrounding a scar to improve circulation, ease pain and promote flexibility; aids healing and rehabilitation

Tear: Split caused by excess force on skin/tissue

UTI: Urinary tract infection

Vagina: Internal passage of a woman's sex organs, birth passage

Vaginal flora: The healthy bacteria that live inside the vagina, dominated by various lactobacillus species, easily unbalanced by synthetic products such as petrochemical-based lube; yet another reason to make sure that if you use lube, it's the organic stuff

Vaginismus: the automatic tightening of the vaginal and pelvic floor muscles in response to attempted vaginal penetration (eg for sex) due to fear. It is an automatic response over which you have no control. May be experienced even if you have previously enjoyed painless penetrative intercourse

Vaginitis: Soreness and swelling inside the vagina

Vulva: The external area, ie what you can see, of a woman's sex organs

Vulvodynia: Chronic pain and discomfort (lasting three months or more) around the opening of the vagina

NOTES

Introduction

1   Barrett et al., "Women's Sexual Health After Childbirth"
2   Barrett et al., "Women's Sexual Health After Childbirth"
3   Shapiro, Gottman and Carrére, "The Baby and the Marriage"; Shapiro, Gottman and Fink, "Short-Term Change in Couples' Conflict"; Cowan and Cowan, *When Partners Become Parents*

Chapter 1: What the Hell is Our Problem?

1   Bennett, "Lie Back and Think of England"; Gathorne-Hardy, *The Rise and Fall of the British Nanny*. The full quote, by Lady Hillingdon (1857–1940) in her 1912 diary entry, was as follows: "When I hear his steps outside my door I lie down on my bed, close my eyes, open my legs and think of England"
2   Lister, Dr Katie, *The Whores of Yore*: I'm sure there were exceptions; however, during most historical periods, contemporary evidence suggests that hopping into bed with your husband was usually some way down the list of fun Saturday-night activities
3   Musacchio, *The Art and Ritual of Childbirth in Renaissance Italy*; Kelly-Gadol, *Did Women Have a Renaissance?*
4   The Independent, "A Brief Cultural History of Sex"
5   Bailey, *Favoured or Oppressed?*
6   The Independent, "A Brief Cultural History of Sex"
7   International Churchill Society, "Lord Randolph's Illness"
8   Emma, *The Mental Load: A Feminist Comic*
9   Waihong, *The Kingdom of Women*
10   Larkin, Phillip, "This Be The Verse"
11   Perry, *The Book You Wish Your Parents Had Read*

Chapter 2: So What Exactly Am I Dealing With?

1 www.heartilyart.com
2 Pethidine Hydrochloride is a synthetic opioid which mimics morphine and is administered during labour for pain relief. Diamorphine is also sometimes administered
3 A method of assisted delivery using a suction cup which attaches to the baby's head. The other end is pulled by the obstetrician
4 A method of assisted delivery using smooth metal tongs (let's be honest, they look like large salad servers) fitting round the baby's head. The handles are pulled by the obstetrician
5 Bump et al., "Assessment of Kegel pelvic muscle exercise performance after brief verbal instruction"
6 NHS, "Overview: Caesarean Section"; Cleveland Clinic, "Cesarean Birth (C-Section)"
7 NHS, "Overview: Postnatal Depression"
8 Rezaie-Keikhaie et al., "Systematic Review and Meta-Analysis of the Prevalence of the Maternity Blues in the Postpartum Period"
9 Office for National Statistics, "Census 2021", www.ons.gov.uk/ peoplepopulationandcommunity/birthsdeathsandmarriages/ livebirths/bulletins/birthsummarytablesenglandandwales/2020
10 VanderKruik et al., "The Global Prevalence of Postpartum Psychosis: A Systematic Review"; Royal College of Psychiatrists, "Postpartum Psychosis"
11 Shapiro and Gottman, "Effects on Marriage of a Psycho-Communicative-Educational Intervention"

Chapter 3: You Want *What*?!

1 Barrett et al., "Women's Sexual Health After Childbirth"
2 Riley, "Starting to Feel Pregnant". These insane figures are based on an average pre-pregnancy uterus size of 7x5x3cm and an average full-term size of 35x25x22cm: that means a shift in volume from 105cm^3 to 19,250cm^3!
3 Not technically 10cm; we use this term to denote the full diameter of the head

4   Jarvis, "How Common is Caesarean Section?"
5   The substance secreted by the mammary glands shortly after the birth, before we start producing breast milk – it's extra-rich in nutrients and antibodies
6   Pelvic floor muscles that are too tight and inflexible, which, confusingly, can have many of the same symptoms as a pelvic floor which needs strengthening
7   Psychology Today, "The Only-Child Family"
8   Sultan, Abdul H. et al, "Pudendal nerve damage during labour: prospective study before and after childbirth", *An International Journal of Obstetrics and Gynaecology*, january 1994, pp22–28

Chapter 4: How About After the Washing Up, Darling?

1   Sims, Karen E. and Meana, Marta, "Why did passion wane? A qualitative study of married women's attributions for declines in sexual desire", *J Sex Marital Ther.* 2010, 36(4), pp360–80, pubmed.ncbi.nlm.nih.gov/20574890/
2   Sawyer, "Esther Perel: 'Fix the Sex and Your Relationship Will Transform'"
3   National Survey of Sexual Attitudes and Lifestyles (Natsal-3)
4   Ahlorg, Tone et al, "Sensual and Sexual Marital Contentment in Parents of Small Children—A Follow-Up Study When the First Child is Four Years Old", *The Journal of Sex Research*, 45(3), August 2008, pp295–304, doi:10.1080/00224490802204423

Chapter 5: The Fatherload

1   Scarff, "Postpartum Depression in Men"
2   Fatherhood Institute, "Fatherhood Institute Research Summary: Fathers and Postnatal Depression"
3   Borneskog et al., "Symptoms of Anxiety and Depression in Lesbian Couples Treated with Donated Sperm: A Descriptive Study"
4   Adair et al., "Cohort Profile: The Cebu Longitudinal Health and Nutrition Survey"; eDrugstore, "Help! I'm a New Father.

What Happened to My Sex Drive?"; Sample, "Becoming a Father Linked to Reduced Testosterone in Men – And Less Sex"

5   Gordon, Zagoory-Sharon, Leckman, "Prolactin, Oxytocin, and the Development of Paternal Behavior across the First Six Months of Fatherhood"

Chapter 6: Take Two

1   That's the hormone for maternal recognition of pregnancy, produced by the trophoblast cells that surround the embryo and which form the placenta after implantation

2   Ayers, S, "Thoughts and emotions during traumatic birth: A qualitative study", *Birth*, 34(3), 2007, pp. 253-263, openaccess.city.ac.uk/id/eprint/2024/

Chapter 7: The Fun Stuff

1   McNish, Hollie, "Conversations with Kids", *Slug*, Little, Brown, 2021

2   Sex Education Forum, "Young People's RSE Poll 2021"

3   Walen, Kim and Elisabeth A. Lloyd, "Female Sexual Arousal: Genital Anatomy and Orgasm in Intercourse" Statistics vary, but only around 25 per cent experience orgasm from penetration alone

4   Male pill: www.marieclaire.co.uk/life/sex-and-relationships/male-pill-coming-68323

5   Ultrasound testicle bath: www.indy100.com/viral/testicle-bath-future-male-contraception-b1937706

RESOURCES BY MEDIUM

&Breathe Resources

- ***Postnatal & Beyond Wellbeing Checklist*** *for six-week check-up and afterwards: www.andbreathewellbeing.com/postnatal-checklist*
- ***Get Your Mojo Back*** *resources website with lots of videos, how-tos and more: www.andbreathewellbeing.com/get-your-mojo-back*

Books & Articles

Barnett, Emma, *Period: It's About Bloody Time*, HQ, 2019

Brathwaite, Candice, *I Am Not Your Baby Mother*, Quercus, 2020

Bushe, Fran, *My Broken Vagina*, Hodder & Stoughton, 2021

Cambridge Women's Pornography Cooperative, *Porn for New Mums*, Chronicle Books, 2008

Clark-Coates, Zoë, *Pregnancy after Loss*, Orion Spring, 2020

Clark-Coates, Zoë, *The Baby Loss Guide*, Orion Spring, 2019

Dabiri, Emma, *Don't Touch My Hair*, Penguin, 2019

Dunn, Jancee, *How Not to Hate Your Husband after Kids,* Little, Brown and Company, 2017

Forbes, Sarah, *Sex in the Museum*, St. Martin's Press, 2016

Gurney, Dr Karen, *Mind the Gap,* Headline Home, 2020

Hatcher-Moore, Jessica, *After Birth*, Souvenir Press, 2021

Hayes, Anya, *Postnatal Pilates*, Bloomsbury, 2020

Hill, Maisie, *Period Power*, Green Tree, 2019

Hill, Milli, *Give Birth Like a Feminist*, HQ, 2021

Judd, Izzy, *Dare to Dream*, Bantam Press, 2017

Kaur, Rupi, *Milk & Honey*, Andrews McMeel Publishing, 2015

Lee, Natalie, *Feeling Myself,* Ebury Digital, 2022

Light, Alex, *You Are Not a Before Picture*, HarperCollins, 2022

McNish, Hollie, *Nobody Told Me*, Little, Brown, 2016

McNish, Hollie, *Slug*, Little, Brown, 2021

Mintz, Dr Laurie, *Becoming Cliterate*, HarperOne, 2018

Nagoski, Emily, *Come As You Are*, Simon & Schuster, 2015

Perel, Esther, *Mating in Captivity*, HarperCollins, 2006

Perry, Philippa, *The Book You Wish Your Parents Had Read (And Your Children Will Be Glad You Did)*, Penguin Life, 2019

Schiftan, Dania, *Coming Soon*, Greystone Books, 2021

Sebold, Alice, *Lucky*, Scribner, 1999

Svanberg, Dr Emma, *Why Birth Trauma Matters*, Pinter & Martin Ltd, 2019

The Hotbed Collective, *More Orgasms Please*, Square Peg, 2019

Unsworth, Emma Jane, *After the Storm: Postnatal Depression and the Utter Weirdness of New Motherhood*, Profile Books, 2021

Van der Kolk, Bessel, *The Body Keeps the Score*, Penguin, 2015

Vickers, Megan, *Stronger*, Green Tree, 2021

Vopni, Kim, *Your Pelvic Floor*, Watkins Publishing, 2021

Whitehouse, Anna, and Farquharson, Matt, *Where's My Happy Ending?* Bluebird, 2020

Websites & Organisations

Aching Arms (comfort after pregnancy and baby loss): www.achingarms.co.uk

Amanda Savage (physiotherapy): www.propelvic.com

Better Help (therapy advice): www.betterhelp.com

Birth Better (pre- and post-birth support): www.makebirthbetter.org

Birth Trauma Association (supports women suffering from PTSD after birth): www.birthtraumaassociation.org.uk

Caroline Bragg (return to impact/running courses): www.instagram.com/carolinebraggpt

Dr Sarah Duvall (physical rehabilitation information): www.instagram.com/drsarahduvall

Fertility Network UK (for fertility challenges and IVF support): www.fertilitynetworkuk.org

Find a therapist in the UK (via the British Association for Counselling and Psychotherapy): www.bacp.co.uk/search/Therapists

Find a women's health physiotherapist in the UK (via the Pelvic Obstetric & Gynaecological Physiotherapy (POGP)): www.thepogp.co.uk/patients/physiotherapists

Find a women's health physical therapist in the USA: www.aptapelvichealth.org/ptlocator

Get Your Mojo Back resources! www.andbreathewellbeing.com/get-your-mojo-back

Lacey Haynes (sex and relationship coach): www.laceyhaynes.com

Laura Dodsworth (100 Vaginas): www.lauradodsworth.com

Mariposa Trust/Saying Goodbye (for miscarriage and pregnancy/baby loss): www.sayinggoodbye.org

Mummy MOT (postnatal physiotherapy practitioners, UK-wide): www.themummymot.com

My Therapist Online (search for online therapy sessions): www.mytherapistonline.co.uk

Pandas UK (pre- and postnatal depression awareness and support): www.pandasfoundation.org.uk

Rape Crisis (support for victims of rape – search for your local branch here too): www.rapecrisis.org.uk

Relate: The Relationship People (advice and support for couples): www.relate.org.uk

Safeline (support with recovery from sexual violence, and counselling): www.safeline.org.uk

Sands (stillbirth and neonatal death charity): www.sands.org.uk

The Lullaby Trust (research into and support for families affected by SIDS (cot death)): www.lullabytrust.org.uk

The Relationship Place (founded by relationship coach Anna Williamson): www.therelationshipplace.co.uk

The Survivors Trust (online platform for self-help and information): www.thesurvivorstrust.org

Tommy's (research into miscarriage and baby loss, support for loss): www.tommys.org

Interactive

APPS

Between – Private Couples: For when you're worried about someone accidentally reading your sexy messages (ahem, kids)

Desire – Couples Game: A fun way to introduce new sexy suggestions to your partner

Gottman Card Decks, from The Gottman Institute – An easy way to access these conversational and physical card prompts

AUDIO-EROTICA

Dipsea – www.dipseastories.com – A whole gamut of audio-erotica, which means you can fine-tune to your desires, plus skip to the good part (perfect when you're a time-poor parent!)

Emjoy – www.letsemjoy.com – A supportive platform to cultivate and normalise female pleasure with guided sessions and audio-erotica

Ferly – www.weareferly.com – Erotica and sexual wellbeing exercises and guides with a focus on sexual self-care and mindful sensuality

Quinn – www.tryquinn.com – Less polished, more real, intimate excerpts

&Jane – www.andjane.com – Socially sourced positive and diverse erotica told from the female perspective. You can also submit stories yourself and follow individual storytellers for their new content

COURSES

How to Not Let Having Kids Ruin Your Sex Life – Workshop by Dr Karen Gurney and The Havelock Clinic: havelockonlineworkshops. teachable.com/p/good-sex-for-new-parents

The Gottman Institute – The Transition to Parenthood gottman. com/product/the-transition-to-parenthood

FEMALE-LED AND MINDFUL SEX TOYS

Dame – www.dameproducts.com – Beautifully made, female-focused toys

Sh! Women's Store – www.sh-womenstore.com – Curated, lovely sex toys for a wide range of tastes

The Natural Love Company – www.thenaturallovecompany.com – Natural and organic products and toys

Vush – uk.vushstimulation.com – Fun brand that promotes loving yourself

FEMINIST AND ETHICAL PORN

Anna Richards – www.frolicme.com – Makes beautiful films and photograph sets

Erika Lust – www.erikalust.com – Award-winning film-maker and feminist porn champion

Make Love Not Porn – www.makelovenotporn.tv – An excellent real-world sex platform run by Cindy Gallop which promotes knowing the difference between porn and real-life intimacy and educates on the topic

O'Actually – www.oactually.com – A curated site that's a great place to start

Sssh – www.sssh.com – This site run by Angie Rowntree hosts crowd-sourced films inspired by members' fantasies and desires

GAMES

'Connect' by The School of Life: www.theschooloflife.com

'The And' by The Skin Deep: www.theskindeep.co.uk/products/the-and-card-game

Vertellis: www.vertellis.com

MINDFULNESS APPS

Calm: www.calm.com

Clementine: www.clementineapp.co.uk

Headspace: www.headspace.com/headspace-meditation-app

Nourish: www.thenourishapp.com

10% Happier: www.tenpercent.com

PEOPLE TO FOLLOW

*@afrosexology_* – A safe space for black people to discuss sexual exploration and liberation

@alexlight_ldn – Alex Light

@alixfox – Joyful sex writer and broadcaster, script consultant for Netflix series *Sex Education*

@andbreathewellbeing – Me!

@danaemercer – Danae Mercer

@froeticsexology – Mindful sex coach

@hannahwitton – Sex education enthusiast

@itscliowood – Also me!

@karleyslutever – Writer and columnist on sex

@lexxsexdoc – Couples clinician helping to reduce conflict and sexual shame

@lunamatatas – 30+ pleasure and confidence

@rubyrare – Queer and silly and really knows her/their stuff

@sexpositive_families – Helping us raise sexually healthy children

@stylemesunday – Natalie Lee

Podcasts

Breaking Mum & Dad – Award-winning author Anna Williamson chats openly and honestly with guests about parenthood and maternal and paternal mental health

Dirty Mother Pukka – Anna Whitehouse talks openly to her guests about sex, relationships, parenthood and more

Doing It! by Hannah Witton – All things sex, relationships, dating and bodies

Lacey & Flynn Have Sex – A couple who now love sex but didn't used to, and how they got to where they are, navigating a ten-year relationship and kids along the way

Motherkind – Zoe Blaskey discusses motherhood from a self-empowerment perspective with leading experts

Sex with Emily – Dr Emily Morse talks about sex and relationships

The Hotbed – Funny, frank and non-cringey sex chat from three women who happen to be mums

The Parent Hood – Marina Fogle and Dr Chiara Hunt answer parents' questions on how to bring up children of all ages

Where Should We Begin by Esther Perel – One of my favourite psychotherapists explores the dynamics of different couples in her enlightening, informative and reassuring podcast

RESOURCES BY CHAPTER

Chapter 1: What the Hell is Our Problem?

Barnett, Emma, *Period*, HQ, 2019

Brathwaite, Candice, *I Am Not Your Baby Mother*, Quercus, 2020

Dabiri, Emma, *Don't Touch My Hair*, Penguin, 2019

Forbes, Sarah, *Sex in the Museum*, St. Martin's Press, 2016

Hill, Maisie, *Period Power*, Green Tree, 2019

Hill, Milli, *Give Birth Like a Feminist*, HQ, 2021

Lee, Natalie, *Feeling Myself*, Ebury Digital, 2022

Light, Alex, *You Are Not a Before Picture*, HarperCollins, 2022

McNish, Hollie, *Slug*, Little, Brown, 20221

Nagoski, Emily, *Come As You Are*, Simon & Schuster, 2015

Perry, Philippa, *The Book You Wish Your Parents Had Read (And Your Children Will Be Glad You Did)*, Penguin Life, 2019

Chapter 2 : So What Exactly Am I Dealing With?

Bushe, Fran, *My Broken Vagina*, Hodder & Stoughton, 2021

Hatcher-Moore, Jessica, *After Birth*, Souvenir Press, 2021

Hayes, Anya, *Postnatal Pilates*, Bloomsbury, 2020

McNish, Hollie, *Nobody Told Me*, Little, Brown, 2016

Svanberg, Dr Emma, *Why Birth Trauma Matters*, Pinter & Martin Ltd, 2019

Unsworth, Emma Jane, *After the Storm*, Profile Books, 2021

Vickers, Megan, *Stronger*, Green Tree, 2021

Vopni, Kim, *Your Pelvic Floor*, Watkins Publishing, 2021

EXERCISES TO TRY

See www.andbreathewellbeing.com/get-your-mojo-back for more information and videos on:

DRA (diastasis rectus abdominus) diagnosis and recovery

Pelvic floor exercises, stretches and proper form

Scar tissue and massage

Functional fitness exercises

Expert guidance and workshops from our contributors

Chapter 3: You Want to *What?!*

Check out other people's vulvas (not ones you know, unless that's your mutual vibe). Getting to know and normalise the myriad shape, sizes, shades of vulvas – as well as the different levels of hirsuteness and more – can be a powerful lesson in acceptance

100 Vaginas: Out of the 100 she photographed as part of the project, writer and photographer Laura Dodsworth interviews 18 women about their vulvas and how these have shaped their lives in an award-winning TV documentary: www.lauradodsworth.com/100-vaginas

Look into pussy gazing: Yep, you read that right. Don't worry, this isn't a group setting thing – well, it is, but not for the actual gazing bit. Lacey Haynes (www.laceyhaynes.com) and other practitioners believe that a lot of our feminine power comes from our vulva and vagina, so understanding how you relate to it and the experiences you have with it can really impact your wellbeing

FITNESS AND RETURNING TO EXERCISE

See www.andbreathewellbeing.com/personal-trainers

Search for your local pre-/postnatally experienced (not just qualified!) fitness trainer

Brianna Battles – www.briannabattles.com

MumHood – www.moveyourframe.com/mumhood

Mutu System – www.mutusystem.com

Rehabilitation – Dr Sarah Duvall – www.instagram.com/drsarahduvall

Return to Impact/Running courses – Caroline Bragg – www.instagram.com/carolinebraggpt

MENTAL HEALTH

Better Help (therapy advice): www.betterhelp.com

Birth Better: www.makebirthbetter.org

Birth Trauma Association: www.birthtraumaassociation.org.uk

Pandas UK (pre- and postnatal depression awareness and support): www.pandasfoundation.org.uk

Find a UK therapist (via the British Association for Counselling and Psychotherapy): www.bacp.co.uk/search/Therapists

MINDFULNESS AND MEDITATION FOR MENTAL HEALTH

Calm: www.calm.com
Clementine: www.clementineapp.co.uk
Headspace: www.headspace.com/headspace-meditation-app
Nourish: www.thenourishapp.com
10% Happier: www.tenpercent.com

PHYSIOTHERAPY/PHYSICAL THERAPY

More recommended physiotherapists can be found on andbreathewellbeing.com/pelvic-floor-physios"
Amanda Savage (physiotherapy): www.propelvic.com
Find a women's health physiotherapist in the UK: www.thepogp.co.uk/patients/physiotherapists
Find a women's health physical therapist in the USA: www.aptapelvichealth.org/ptlocator

Chapter 4: How About After the Washing Up, Darling?

Cambridge Women's Pornography Cooperative, *Porn for New Mums*, Chronicle Books, 2008
Gurney, Dr Karen, *Mind the Gap*, Headline Home, 2020
Perel, Esther, *Mating in Captivity*, HarperCollins, 2006
The Hotbed Collective, *More Orgasms Please*, Square Peg, 2019

MENTAL HEALTH

Relate: The Relationship People (advice and support for couples): www.relate.org.uk
The Relationship Place (founded by relationship coach Anna Williamson): www.therelationshipplace.co.uk
It's also possible to find some brilliant psychotherapists and counsellors online at places like My Therapist Online (www.mytherapistonline.co.uk) and Better Help (www.betterhelp.

com), or simply by Googling a therapist near you. It's okay to try a session or two first before finding the right therapist for you or you and your partner

Chapter 5: The Fatherload

Dunn, Jancee, *How Not to Hate Your Husband after Kids*, Little, Brown and Company, 2017

Perel, Esther, *Mating in Captivity*, Hodder & Stoughton, 2007

Whitehouse, Anna, and Farquharson, Matt, *Where's My Happy Ending?* Bluebird, 2020

EXERCISES TO TRY

These no-pressure card games are a great place to start to connect with your other half and deepen the conversation and honesty.

'Connect' by The School of Life: www.theschooloflife.com

'The And' by The Skin Deep: www.theskindeep.co.uk/products/the-and-card-game

Vertellis: www.vertellis.com

If you want to explore further, the brilliant Dr Karen Gurney has this online course available too:

How to Not Let Having Kids Ruin Your Sex Life – Workshop by Dr Karen Gurney: havelockonlineworkshops.teachable.com/p/good-sex-for-new-parents

Chapter 6: Take Two

Clark-Coates, Zoë, *Pregnancy after Loss*, Orion Spring, 2020

Clark-Coates, Zoë, *The Baby Loss Guide*, Orion Spring, 2019

Haslett, Emma & Griffith, Gabby, *Big Fat Negative*, Hachette, 2022

Judd, Izzy, *Dare to Dream*, Bantam Press, 2017

Kaur, Rupi, *Milk & Honey*, Andrews McMeel Publishing, 2015

Sebold, Alice, *Lucky*, Scribner, 1999

Van der Kolk, Bessel, *The Body Keeps the Score*, Penguin, 2015

FERTILITY

Big Fat Negative Podcast www.bigfatnegative.com

Fertility Network UK (for fertility challenges and IVF support): www.fertilitynetworkuk.org

LOSS
Aching Arms (comfort after pregnancy and baby loss): www.achingarms.co.uk

Mariposa Trust/Saying Goodbye (for miscarriage and pregnancy/ baby loss): www.sayinggoodbye.org

Sands (stillbirth and neonatal death charity): www.sands.org.uk

The Lullaby Trust (research into and support for families affected by SIDS (cot death)): www.lullabytrust.org.uk

Tommy's (research into miscarriage and baby loss, support for loss): www.tommys.org

SEXUAL ASSAULT AND RAPE
Rape Crisis (support for victims of rape – search for your local branch here too): www.rapecrisis.org.uk

Safeline (support with recovery from sexual violence, and counselling): www.safeline.org.uk

The Survivors Trust (online platform for self-help and information): www.thesurvivorstrust.org

Chapter 7: The Fun Stuff
Gurney, Dr Karen, *Mind the Gap*, Headline Home, 2020

Mintz, Dr Laurie, *Becoming Cliterate*, HarperOne, 2018

Nagoski, Emily, *Come As You Are*, Simon & Schuster, 2015

Schiftan, Dania, *Coming Soon*, Greystone Books, 2021

The Hotbed Collective, *More Orgasms Please*, Square Peg, 2019

www.self.com/story/this-is-why-you-should-pay-for-porn

APPS & GAMES
A Year of Dates: www.ayearofdates.co.uk

Between – Private Couples: For when you're worried about someone accidentally reading your sexy messages

Desire – Couples Game: A fun way to introduce new sexy suggestions to your partner

Gottman Card Decks, from The Gottman Institute: An easy way to access these conversational and physical card prompts

AUDIO-EROTICA

Dipsea – www.dipseastories.com – A whole gamut of audio-erotica, which means you can fine-tune to your desires, plus skip to the good part (perfect when you're a time-poor parent!)

Emjoy – www.letsemjoy.com – A supportive platform to cultivate and normalise female pleasure with guided sessions and audio-erotica

Ferly – www.weareferly.com – Erotica and sexual wellbeing exercises and guides with a focus on sexual self-care and mindful sensuality

Quinn – www.tryquinn.com – Less polished, more real, intimate excerpts

&Jane – www.andjane.com – Socially sourced positive and diverse erotica told from the female perspective. You can also submit stories yourself and follow individual storytellers for their new content

FEMALE-LED AND MINDFUL SEX TOYS

Dame – www.dameproducts.com – Beautifully made, female-focused toys

Sh! Women's Store – www.sh-womenstore.com – Curated, lovely sex toys for a wide range of tastes

The Natural Love Company – www.thenaturallovecompany.com – Natural and organic products and toys

Vush – uk.vushstimulation.com – Fun brand that promotes loving loving yourself

FEMINIST AND ETHICAL PORN

Anna Richards – www.frolicme.com – Makes beautiful films and photograph sets

Erika Lust – www.erikalust.com – Award-winning film-maker and feminist porn champion

Make Love Not Porn – www.makelovenotporn.tv – An excellent real-world sex platform run by Cindy Gallop which promotes knowing the difference between porn and real-life intimacy and educates on the topic

O'Actually – www.oactually.com – A curated site that's a great place to start

Sssh – www.sssh.com – This site run by Angie Rowntree hosts crowd-sourced films inspired by members' fantasies and desires

ORGANIC AND ETHICAL LUBRICATION AND CONDOMS

Hanx – www.hanxofficial.com

Sustain Natural – www.sustainnatural.com

Fairsquared – www.fairsquared.info/fairtrade-products-en/condoms-en

YES Organics – Water-based (condom-friendly), oil-based, anal or vaginal moisturisers, all organic. What more could you ask? – www.yesyesyes.org

Coconut oil, almond oil and any other naturally derived oils are also great for scar massage – but do not use with condoms!

PODCASTS

Big Fat Negative Podcast – the podcast about IVF and infertility. Co-hosted by journalists Emma and Gabriella, the show follows their stories and interviews a range of experts on the not-so-simple journey to motherhood.

Breaking Mum & Dad – Award-winning author Anna Williamson chats openly and honestly with guests about parenthood and maternal and paternal mental health

Dirty Mother Pukka – Anna Whitehouse talks openly to her guests about sex, relationships, parenthood and more

Doing It! by Hannah Witton – All things sex, relationships, dating and bodies

Lacey & Flynn Have Sex – A couple who now love sex but didn't used to, and how they got to where they are, navigating a ten-year relationship and kids along the way

Motherkind – Zoe Blaskey discusses motherhood from a self-empowerment perspective with leading experts

Sex with Emily by Dr Emily Morse – Sex, relationships and answers to listener questions

The Hotbed – Funny, frank and non-cringey sex chat from three women who happen to be mums

The Parent Hood – Marina Fogle and Dr Chiara Hunt answer parents' questions on how to bring up children of all ages

The Sexual Wellness Sessions – A series of interviews hosted by psychosexual and relationship therapist, Dr Kate Moyle.

Where Should We Begin – Esther Perel explores the dynamics of different couples in her enlightening and reassuring podcast

SEX-POSITIVE ACCOUNTS

*@afrosexology_* – A safe space for black people to discuss sexual exploration and liberation

@alixfox – Joyful sex writer and broadcaster, script consultant for Netflix series *Sex Education*

@alexlight_ldn – Brilliant body confidence campaigner helping women feel better about their bodies

@froeticsexology – Mindful sex coach

@hannahwitton – Sex education enthusiast

@karleyslutever – Writer and columnist on sex

@lexxsexdoc – Couples clinician helping to reduce conflict and sexual shame

@lunamatatas – 30+ pleasure and confidence

@rubyrare – Queer and silly and really knows her/their stuff

@sexpositive_families – Helping us raise sexually healthy children

BIBLIOGRAPHY

All the resource books listed above, as well as:

Adair, Linda S., et al., "Cohort Profile: The Cebu Longitudinal Health and Nutrition Survey", *International Journal of Epidemiology*, 40 (3), 619–25 (2011)

Al-Gailani, Salim, and Davis, Angela, "Introduction to 'Transforming Pregnancy Since 1900'", *Studies in History and Philosophy of Science Part B*, 47, 229–32 (2014)

Backhouse, Constance, "Review: Marriage, Women, and Property: A Legal History of Enforced Dependence", Cambridge University Press, 2018. www.cambridge.org/core/journals/american-bar-foundation-research-journal/article/abs/marriage-women-and-property-a-legal-history-of-enforced-dependence/24B193AF1196004CCC6B7E942524C628

Bailey, Joanne, *Favoured or Oppressed? Married Women, Property and "Coverture" in England, 1660–1800*, Cambridge University Press, 2003

Barrett, Geraldine, et al., "Women's Sexual Health after Childbirth", *BJOG*, 107 (2), 186–95 (2000)

Bennett, Oliver, "Lie Back and Think of England", *The Independent*, Sunday, 21 January 1996. www.independent.co.uk/life-style/lie-back-and-think-of-england-1324969.html

Borneskog, Catrin et al, "Symptoms of Anxiety and Depression in Lesbian Couples Treated with Donated Sperm: A Descriptive Study", *BJOG*, 120 (7), 839–46 (2013). doi.org/10.1111/1471-0528.12214

Braekken, Ingeborg H. et al, "Can Pelvic Floor Muscle Training Improve Sexual Function in Women with Pelvic Organ Prolapse? A Randomized Controlled Trial", *The Journal of Sexual Medicine*, 12 (2), 470–80 (2015)

Brittle, Zach, "When Three's Not the Charm: How to Manage the Higher Risk of Divorce When Baby Comes Along", *The Washington Post*, 30 June 2015. www.washingtonpost.com/news/inspired-life/wp/2015/06/30/when-threes-not-the-charm-how-to-manage-the-higher-risk-of-divorce-when-baby-comes-along/

Bump, Richard C et al, "Assessment of Kegel Pelvic Muscle Exercise Performance after Brief Verbal Instruction", *American Journal of Obstetrics and Gynecology*, 165 (2), 322–9 (1991)

Carlini, Denise, and Davidman, Ann, *Motherhood – Is It for Me? Your Step-by-Step Guide to Clarity*, Transformation Books, 2016

Centre of Perinatal Excellence (COPE), "Postnatal Rage". www.cope.org.au/new-parents/first-weeks/postpartum-rage/

Cleveland Clinic, "Cesarean Birth (C-Section)". www.nhs.uk/conditions/caesarean-section/

Cowan, C. P., and Cowan, P. A., *When Partners Become Parents*, Lawrence Erlbaum Associates Publishers, 2000

Curtis, Scarlett, *Feminists Don't Wear Pink and Other Lies*, Penguin, 2018

DeGrazia, Victoria, with Furlough, Ellen (eds), *The Sex of Things*, University of California Press, 1996

De Pietro, MaryAnn, "What Happens When Estrogen Levels Are Low?" *Medical News Today*, 27 February 2018. www.medicalnewstoday.com/articles/321064

Dingfelder, Sadie, "Must Babies Always Breed Marital Discontent?" *Monitor on Psychology*, 42 (3), 51 (2011)

Doss, Brian, and Rhoades, Galena, "The Transition to Parenthood: Impact on Couples' Romantic Relationships", *Current Opinion in Psychology*, 13, 25–8 (2017)

eDrugstore, "Help! I'm a New Father. What Happened to My Sex Drive?" 30 July 2021. www.edrugstore.com/blog/erectile-dysfunction/help-im-a-new-father-what-happened-to-my-sex-drive/

Emma, *The Mental Load*, Murdoch Books, 2018

Espin, Oliva M., "Cultural and Historical Influences on Sexuality in Hispanic/Latin Women: Implications for Psychotherapy", in O. Espin, *Latina Realities: Essays on Healing, Migration and Sexuality*, 83–96, Routledge, New York, 2019

Fatherhood Institute, "Fatherhood Institute Research Summary: Fathers and Postnatal Depression", 10 September 2018. www.fatherhoodinstitute.org/2018/fatherhood-institute-research-summary-fathers-and-postnatal-depression/

Geddes, Linda, "Why the Truth about Breastfeeding and Weight Loss Is Far from the Myth", *The Guardian*, 2 July 2018, www.theguardian.com/lifeandstyle/shortcuts/2018/jul/02/truth-about-breastfeeding-weight-loss-myth-serena-williams

Gordon, Ilanit, Zagoory-Sharon, Orna, and Leckman, James F., "Prolactin, Oxytocin, and the Development of Paternal Behavior across the First Six Months of Fatherhood", *Hormones and Behavior*, 58 (3), 513–18 (2010)

Green, Lucinda, "Postnatal Depression", *Royal College of Psychiatrists*, 2018. www.rcpsych.ac.uk/mental-health/problems-disorders/post-natal-depression

Grose, Jessica, "Fighting Constantly After Baby? Read This", *The New York Times*, 8 May 2020. www.nytimes.com/article/fighting-after-baby-guide.html

Hendrick, V., Altshuler, L. L. and Suri, R., "Hormonal Changes in the Postpartum and Implications for Postpartum Depression", *Psychosomatics*, 39 (2), 93–101 (1998)

History Extra, "A Brief History of Sex and Sexuality in Ancient Greece", 22 September 2021. www.historyextra.com/period/ancient-greece/a-brief-history-of-sex-and-sexuality-in-ancient-greece/

HSE.ie, "Postnatal Depression – Causes". www2.hse.ie/conditions/mental-health/postnatal-depression/causes-of-postnatal-depression.html

Ibrahim, Hanna, "Almost Half of Women in the UK Have a Sexual Health Problem. So Why Aren't We Talking about It?" *Stylist Magazine*, 15 April 2020. www.stylist.co.uk/beauty/sexual-health-wellness-tips-mind-body-contraception-sex-relationships/363429

International Churchill Society, "Lord Randolph's Illness", January 2020. winstonchurchill.org/publications/churchill-bulletin/bulletin-163-jan-2022/lord-randolphs-illness/

Jarvis, Sarah, "How Common Is Caesarean Section", *Patient.info*, 13 April 2021. patient.info/pregnancy/labour-childbirth/caesarean-section#nav-6

Kelly-Gadol, Joan, *Did Women Have a Renaissance?* Reprinted from R. Bridenthai and C. Koonz (eds), *Becoming Visible*, 137–64, Houghton Mifflin Co, 1977

Lady Hillingdon (1857–1940) in S. Ratcliffe (ed.), *Oxford Essential Quotations* (4th ed.), as quoted in J. Gathorne-Hardy, *The Rise and Fall of the British Nanny*, The Dial Press, 1972

Larkin, Phillip, "This Be The Verse", *Poetry Foundation*. www.poetryfoundation.org/poems/48419/this-be-the-verse

Mayor, S., "Sixty Seconds on . . . Tokophobia", *British Medical Journal*, 362: k3933 (2018)

MedlinePlus, "Managing Your Weight Gain during Pregnancy", updated 5 October 2022. www.medlineplus.gov/ency/patientinstructions/000603.htm

Moussawi, Ghassan, and Patil, Vrushali, "Race and Sexuality", in L. Spillman (ed.), *Oxford Bibliographies in Sociology*, Oxford University Press, Oxford, 2020. www.oxfordbibliographies.com/view/document/obo-9780199756384/obo-9780199756384-0247.xml

Musacchio, Jacqueline, *The Art and Ritual of Childbirth in Renaissance Italy*, Yale University Press, 1999

National Childbirth Trust (NCT), "Postnatal Depression in Dads: 10 Things You Should Know", 17 October 2021, www.nct.org.uk/life-parent/emotions/postnatal-depression-dads-10-things-you-should-know

NHS, "Overview: Caesarean Section". www.nhs.uk/conditions/caesarean-section/

NHS, "Overview: Postnatal Depression". www.nhs.uk/mental-health/conditions/post-natal-depression/overview/

NHS Digital, "Maternity Services Monthly Statistics, September 2021, Experimental Statistics", 16 December 2021. digital.nhs.

uk/data-and-information/publications/statistical/maternity-services-monthly-statistics/september-2021-experimental-statistics

Office for National Statistics, "Census 2021", www.ons.gov.uk/peoplepopulationandcommunity/birthsdeathsandmarriages/livebirths/bulletins/birthsummarytablesenglandandwales/2020

Psychology Today, "The Only-Child Family" www.psychologytoday.com/us/basics/family-dynamics/only-child-family

Relate, "Top 4 Reasons Couples Argue after Having a Baby". www.relate.org.uk/relationship-help/help-family-life-and-parenting/new-parents/top-4-reasons-couples-argue-after-having-baby

Rezaie-Keikhaie, Khadije et al, "Systematic Review and Meta-Analysis of the Prevalence of the Maternity Blues in the Postpartum Period", *Journal of Obstetric, Gynecologic and Neonatal Nursing*, 49 (2), 127–36 (2020). doi.org/10.1016/j.jogn.2020.01.001

Riley, Laura, "Starting to Feel Pregnant", *Parents*. www.parents.com/pregnancy/week-by-week/7/starting-to-feel-pregnant/

Roberts, Dorothy, *Killing the Black Body: Race, Reproduction, and the Meaning of Liberty*, Vintage UK, 1999

Royal College of Psychiatrists, "Postpartum Psychosis". www.rcpsych.ac.uk/mental-health/problems-disorders/postpartum-psychosis

Sacomori, Cinara, and Cardoso, Fernando Luiz, "Predictors of Improvement in Sexual Function of Women with Urinary Incontinence after Treatment with Pelvic Floor Exercises: A Secondary Analysis", *The Journal of Sexual Medicine*, 12 (3), 746–55 (2015)

Sample, Ian, "Becoming a Father Linked to Reduced Testosterone in Men – And Less Sex", *The Guardian*, Friday, 14 February 2014. www.theguardian.com/science/2014/feb/14/father-reduced-testosterone-men-sex

Sawyer, Miranda, "Esther Perel: 'Fix the Sex and Your Relationship Will Transform'", *The Guardian*, 30 September 2018. www.

theguardian.com/lifeandstyle/2018/sep/30/esther-perel-fix-the-sex-and-your-relationship-will-transform-esther-perel

Scarff, J. R., "Postpartum Depression in Men", *Innovations in Clinical Neuroscience*, 16 (5–6): 11–14 (2019). www.ncbi.nlm.nih.gov/pmc/articles/PMC6659987/

Schiedel, Bonnie, "17 Mind-Blowing Ways Your Body Changes after Giving Birth", *Today's Parent*, 9 May 2018. www.todaysparent.com/baby/postpartum-care/mind-blowing-ways-your-body-changes-after-giving-birth/

Sex Education Forum, "Young People's RSE Poll 2021", February 2022. www.sexeducationforum.org.uk/sites/default/files/field/attachment/Young%20Peoples%20RSE%20Poll%202021%20-%20SEF%201%20Feb%202022.pdf

Shapiro, Alyson F., and Gottman, John M., "Effects on Marriage of a Psycho-Communicative-Educational Intervention with Couples Undergoing the Transition to Parenthood, Evaluation at 1-Year Post Intervention", *Journal of Family Communication*, 5 (1), 1–24 (2005)

Shapiro, Alyson F. et al, "The Baby and the Marriage: Identifying factors that Buffer against Decline in Marital Satisfaction after the First Baby Arrives", *Journal of Family Psychology*, 14 (1), 59–70 (2000). doi.org/10.1037/0893-3200.14.1.59

Shapiro, Alyson F., Gottman, John M., and Fink, Brandi, "Short-Term Change in Couples' Conflict Following a Transition to Parenthood Intervention", *Couple and Family Psychology*, 4 (4), 239–51 (2015)

Stechyson, Natalie, "Why Do I Hate My Partner after Having A Baby? Life after Birth" *Huffington Post*, 6 June 2019. www.huffingtonpost.co.uk/entry/hate-partner-after-having-baby_l_610874fae4b0497e67026c50

Sultan, Abdul H. et al, "Pudendal nerve damage during labour: prospective study before and after childbirth", *An International Journal of Obstetrics and Gynaecology*, january 1994, pp22–28

The Independent, "A Brief Cultural History of Sex", 23 September 2008. www.independent.co.uk/life-style/love-sex/culture-of-love/a-brief-cultural-history-of-sex-938527.html

Van Anders, Sari M., Hipp, Lauren E. and Kane Low, Lisa, "Exploring Co-Parent Experiences of Sexuality in the First 3 Months after Birth", *The Journal of Sexual Medicine*, 10 (8), 1988–99 (2013)

VanderKruik, Rachel et al, "The Global Prevalence of Postpartum Psychosis: A Systematic Review", *BMC Psychiatry*, 17 (1) (2017). doi.org/10.1186/s12888-017-1427-7

Vidal-Ortiz, Salvador, Robinson, Brandon Andrew, and Khan, Cristina, *Race and Sexuality*, Polity Press, 2018

Waihong, Choo, *The Kingdom of Women*, I. B. Tauris, 2017

Whipps, Heather, "A Brief History of Human Sex", *Live Science*, 27 July 2006. www.livescience.com/7088-history-human-sex.html

Zenhausern, Alissia, "Your Postpartum Hormone Timeline: Here's What Happens", *Hello Postpartum*, 22 July 2020. hellopostpartum.com/postpartum-hormone-timeline/

ACKNOWLEDGEMENTS

This book was a long time in the making (aren't they all?), not least because it was inspired by the journey I've been on, and slowed by a global pandemic, business crisis, hyperemesis-riddled pregnancy, new baby, house move, full renovation and therapy by the truckload.

So hats off to my amazing family and friends who've been so supportive along the way: Bryn, my wonderful husband whose patience knows no bounds; my daughters, Delphi and Echo who are both the reason behind the book and who bring me joy every day. My friends (especially Cee, Caroline, Adele and Jo) and family (Loong, Kay and my crazy parents).

Heartfelt thanks to all the health professionals who've helped me along the way: Amanda Savage; therapists Jonathan Pease, Hannah Taylor, Christine Usher and Emily Dixon; Anna Clarkson; Caroline Bragg (again); the team at Fix London. And thank you to the NHS staff at Homerton University Hospital, Newham University Hospital and Princess Alexandra Hospital for my maternity, perinatal mental health and ectopic surgery care, particularly Gitty Blum, Kate Mayers and my midwife, Victoria.

I'm hugely appreciative of the time taken by my incredible contributors: Amanda Savage, Christina Pickworth, Rosalie Genay, Natalie Lee, Sarah Forbes, Alex Kasozi, Lisa Williams, Lavinia and Bryan Winch, Brooke Vandermolen, Emma Svanberg, Sophie Whippy, Hannah Johnson and of course, Bryn. Thank you.

Huge thanks to Emma Barnett, who introduced me to my first editor at *The Telegraph*, Claire Cohen, and set me on the path to writing more intentionally, and to Claire for publishing my first article. Thanks to Anya Hayes for commissioning me and being a fab Insta-friend, and to the whole team at Watkins for all their hard work. Hope I've done ok!